ACCESS Health Press

Checkpoint Inhibitors

A Key to Curing Cancer

William A. Haseltine Ph.D.
And
Amara Thomas

ISBN: 979-8-9890823-9-1 (Digital)
ISBN: 979-8-9921583-0-4 (Paperback)
ISBN: 979-8-9921583-1-1 (Hardcover)

*Some of the stories shared here are true, while others are invented or embellished. However, all of them are rooted in the factual experiences of real individuals. Some narratives have been shortened for clarity. Please note that names and identifying details may have been altered to protect privacy, and certain events may have been condensed.

Cover art & Editing by Kim Hazel

All author proceeds from the sale of this book will be donated to the nonprofit global think tank ACCESS Health International.

Acknowledgments

We thank the ACCESS Health US team, Koloman Rath, Griffin McCombs, and Roberto Patarca, for their support in creating this book.

This work is supported by ACCESS Health International (www.accessh.org).

Dedication

William Haseltine, Ph.D.

To my mentors and friends, you opened the road and were the wind behind me. Thank you for a wonderful life.

Amara Thomas:

To my loving family and friends.

Recent Books by William A. Haseltine

Affordable Excellence: The Singapore Healthcare Story; William A Haseltine (2013)

Improving the Health of Mother and Child: Solutions from India; Priya Anant, Prabal Vikram Singh, Sofi Bergkvist, William A. Haseltine & Anita George (2014)

Modern Aging: A Practical Guide for Developers, Entrepreneurs, and Startups in the Silver Market; Edited by Sofia Widén, Stephanie Treschow, and William A. Haseltine (2015)

Aging with Dignity: Innovation and Challenge is Sweden-The Voice of Care Professionals; Sofia Widen and William A. Haseltine (2017)

Every Second Counts: Saving Two Million Lives. India's Emergency Response System.The EMRI Story; William A Haseltine (2017)

Voices in Dementia Care; Anna Dirksen and William A Haseltine (2018)

Aging Well; Jean Galiana and William A. Haseltine (2019)

World Class. Adversity, Transformation and Success and NYU Langone Health; William A. Haseltine (2019)

A Family Guide to Covid: Questions and Answers for Parents, Grandparents, and Children; William A. Haseltine (2020)

A Covid Back To School Guide: Questions and Answers for Parents and Students; William A. Haseltine (2020)

Covid Commentaries: A Chronicle of a Plague, Volumes I, II, III, IV, V, and VI; William A. Haseltine (2020)

My Lifelong Fight Against Disease: From Polio and AIDS to Covid-19; William A. Haseltine (2020)

Science as a Superpower: My Lifelong Fight Against Disease And The Heroes Who Made It Possible; William A. Haseltine (2021)

Variants!: The Shape-Shifting Challenge of Covid-19 Vaccine Evasion & Reinfection; William A. Haseltine (2021)

Covid Related Post-traumatic Stress Disorder (CV-PTSD): What It Is And What To Do About It; William A. Haseltine (2021)

Natural Immunity And Covid-19: What It Is And How It Can Save Your Life; William A. Haseltine (2022)

Omicron: From Pandemic to Endemic; William A. Haseltine (2022)

Monoclonal Antibodies: The Once and Future Cure for Covid-19; William A. Haseltine and Griffin McCombs (2023)

The Future of Medicine: Healing Yourself: Regenerative Medicine Part One; William A. Haseltine (2023)

Viroids and Virusoids: Nature's Own mRNAs; William A. Haseltine and Koloman Rath (2023)

CAR T: A New Cure for Cancer, Autoimmune and Inherited Disease; William A. Haseltine and Amara Thomas (2023)

Ending Hepatitis C: A Seven-step Plan for a Successful Eradication Program: A Roadmap for Ending Endemic Disease Globally; William A. Haseltine and Kaelyn Varner (2023)

The COVID-19 Textbook: Science, Medicine and Public Health; William A. Haseltine and Roberto Patarca (2023)

Better Eyesight: What You and Modern Medicine Can Do to Improve Your Vision; William A. Haseltine and Kim Hazel (2024)

Molecular Biology of SARS-CoV-2: Opportunities for Antivirus Drug Development; William A. Haseltine and Roberto Patarca (2024)

Fusion! The Melding of Human and Machine Intelligence; William A. Haseltine and Griffin McCombs (2024)

Contents

Introduction

"If we do not give you any treatment, the life expectancy is in the order of months."

Richard Metz, a loving husband, father, and grandfather from Wilton, Connecticut, felt his world crash with these words. A cold numbness spread through him. It wasn't the first time he had faced cancer, but the sense of finality in his doctor's voice was unmistakable.

Richard's first encounter with melanoma came in 2003. Back then, it was a small, seemingly harmless mole on his back. The diagnosis—Stage II melanoma—had been a shock, but surgery had been swift, and the doctors reassured him it hadn't spread to other parts of his body. Richard moved on with his life, grateful to have escaped the worst.

But in 2007, after years of peaceful remission, Richard found himself back in the hospital, this time feeling utterly unwell.

Something was wrong. He couldn't sleep through the night without waking in cold sweats, his body drenched as if it had run a marathon. His energy was draining away, and his liver enzymes were dangerously high. What was happening? No one could have predicted that the innocent-looking mole, removed years earlier, had silently returned with a vengeance. Now, a four-inch tumor pressed against his liver—a Stage IV melanoma.

At that moment, Richard's oncologist, Dr. Harriet Kluger, delivered the grim prognosis—mere months to live. She would never cast such a definitive and dark forecast to patients with Stage IV cancer now, given current breakthroughs in cancer research. But even though options at the time seemed hopelessly limited, Richard wasn't ready to give up. He couldn't. With Dr. Kluger by his side, he faced an impossible choice.

Extensive surgery was the first option to fight the tumor, but at great risk: a 15-20% chance he wouldn't survive the procedure. And even if he did, surgery alone wouldn't be enough. Chemotherapy, the other option, would only buy time against his cancer's relentless advance.

Despite the bleak outlook, Richard and Dr. Kluger refused to surrender. They agreed on a daring plan—surgery followed by an experimental treatment called cancer immunotherapy. Today, immunotherapies are a powerful tool in the fight against cancer, but back in 2007, they were uncharted territory. Scientists were just beginning to unlock the immune system's potential to fight cancer. No one could predict whether it would work or the side effects. But for Richard, it was a chance—a slim one, but a chance nonetheless.

Weeks into the trial, Richard's body began to change in ways he could never have predicted. The treatment added 31 pounds of water weight to his frame almost overnight, transforming him into what his family jokingly called "the Pillsbury Doughboy." But the humor wore off as quickly as the weight dropped. Soon, his skin burned and itched so fiercely that it felt like he'd been rolling in poison ivy. Every new symptom felt like a betrayal—wasn't this supposed to make him better? Meanwhile, the tumor seemed stubbornly unchanged.

Still, Dr. Kluger suspected that immunotherapy was working in ways they couldn't yet measure. After Richard underwent liver surgery, something remarkable happened: while the major tumor had been removed, the smaller lesions in his body stopped growing. "We thought that [the immunotherapy] had not done anything, but in fact once the major tumor was removed, there were other things in the body that did not grow very much or at all after that," she later reflected.

A new sense of hope began to grow in Richard. He traveled more, worked with renewed focus, and cherished time with his family. But just when he thought the worst was behind him, February 2011 brought a fresh wave of dread. An MRI scan revealed a new tumor, this time in his brain.

This kind of recurrence is all too common for melanoma patients. For nearly 50% of people with melanoma, the cancer eventually spreads to the brain, and when it does, the odds are dire. Cancers perched on this delicate organ are notoriously difficult to treat. Richard underwent gamma knife surgery—a misleading name for a precise, concentrated dose of radiation directed at the tumor. The procedure worked, but it wasn't enough. New brain metastases kept appearing. "The brain mets kept popping up," Richard recalled. "In one month, I had eight treated by gamma knife."

For years, Richard cycled through treatment options, enduring a grueling dance between shock and relief. But in 2014, the tides finally began to turn. He joined a clinical trial for a new class of immunotherapy drugs: ***checkpoint inhibitors.***

Checkpoint inhibitors were a bold, novel approach to cancer treatment. Unlike earlier therapies, these drugs unleashed the body's own immune system to recognize and attack cancer cells. The specific drug Richard was given, Keytruda, had shown promise but had not yet been tested on patients with brain metastases.

Richard received a high-strength version of the drug, and though his body initially struggled with adverse effects, a lower, FDA-approved dosage brought miraculous results: his cancer stabilized, and Richard's life regained a fragile equilibrium.

After years of battling the odds, Richard's life now has a rhythm again—one no longer defined by hospital visits or life-or-death decisions. Checkpoint inhibitors didn't just give him time, they gave him back his purpose. Whether spending time with his growing family or mentoring others facing their cancer journeys, Richard is living proof of what modern medicine can achieve. And he continues his fight not just for himself, but for the future of everyone touched by cancer as a patient advocate.

Richard Metz's story is not just a personal tale of survival; it reflects the remarkable transformation that immunotherapies, particularly checkpoint inhibitors, have brought to cancer care over the last two decades. Cancer is unpredictable, relentless, and deeply personal. But thanks to groundbreaking advances like checkpoint inhibitors, we now have powerful allies in the fight against this disease. For Richard, they restored a semblance of normalcy after years of uncertainty, proving that even in the darkest moments, hope is possible.

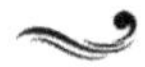

This book is not only for those curious about the future of cancer care, it's for anyone touched by this illness—for patients, caregivers, friends, and loved ones. You might find yourself feeling overwhelmed, as Richard did. Cancer changes everything. However, being well informed about your condition and the treatment options available can help you regain a sense of control in the midst of uncertainty. Reading this book might even save your life.

Checkpoint inhibitors, the central focus of this book, represent a breakthrough in cancer therapy. They have transformed the treatment of several cancers—melanoma, lung cancer, kidney cancer, and more—and could offer life-changing hope for you or someone you care about. These drugs are not the final answer in our search to cure cancer, but they are a monumental step forward in the fight.

As someone who has spent a lifetime studying cancer, I have seen firsthand how the science of this disease has evolved. In the 1990s, I helped establish the Division of Cancer Pharmacology at the Dana-Farber Cancer Institute, where I worked alongside world-class oncologists and researchers to develop new therapies. Over the years, I have taught at Harvard, mentored future cancer researchers, and collaborated with biotech companies to bring innovative drugs to patients. I've seen the triumphs and the heartbreaking setbacks, but one thing is clear—science is steadily pushing forward, and treatments like checkpoint inhibitors are part of that wave of progress.

As you read on, my hope is that this book will serve as a guide for you on this journey—whether you're a patient, a caregiver, or simply someone trying to understand the latest advances in cancer therapy. You'll find a mix of scientific insight, real-life stories, and practical information to help you navigate the complex world of cancer treatment. Together, we'll explore what checkpoint inhibitors are, how they work, and why they may hold the key to a new era ofcancer care.

PART I

Cancer, The Story We All Share

CHAPTER 1

What is Cancer?

Everyone knows of cancer. Most of us have felt it's presence, whether through personal experience or watching a loved one struggle. Surprisingly, although the illness has accompanied humankind for as long as we have lived, the quest to understand cancer—and adequately address it—has only made significant progress in the last century.

Cancer is so difficult to pinpoint because of its sheer diversity. The term "cancer" is an umbrella that covers over one hundred distinct diseases, each as unique as the tissues they arise from. Lung cancer, for instance, bears little resemblance to breast cancer or blood-borne cancers like leukemia.

For some people, cancer creeps slowly, gradually taking over the body; for others, it infiltrates aggressively in mere weeks. As we've seen with Richard Metz, it can start in one place—the skin, the tongue, the blood, the lungs, anywhere—only to reappear elsewhere. Categorizing and responding to this vast array of cancer types was an immense challenge, especially before the advent of modern diagnostic technologies.

With time, scientists have found the link between these seemingly unrelated symptoms. The cause of cancers is actually something very ordinary; it's a process that occurs in everyone every single day: DNA mutations, or genetic changes in our cells.

Let's put these mutations into context. Picture a metropolis of staggering proportions, a cellular city with over 37 trillion inhabitants. Every building, road, and park represents different organs and tissues working together to keep everything running smoothly. The trillions of workers in this city are your cells, performing specific tasks to maintain order and function. New workers are trained and replace the older ones when they retire. Everything follows a blueprint—the DNA—guiding how each worker operates.

These genetic blueprints aren't perfect. There are over three billion letters in this manual. Now imagine copying this manual every time your cells divide to create a new cell. It's bound to result in a few "spelling errors"—or mutations—along the way. These mutations form *all of the time*. It's so inevitable that, even now as you read this passage, there are undoubtedly cells randomly creating DNA changes in your body. Still, this cannot be overlooked: exposure to certain environmental factors, such as tobacco smoke, ultraviolet radiation from the sun, or even certain viruses, can also trigger genetic mutations. These exposures are called carcinogens, and preventing exposure to these factors lessens the chance of getting cancer.

So what happens when errors appear in our DNA? For the most part, nothing. Most DNA mutations are harmless. In many cases, our cellular workers can still understand and follow these blueprints, just as you can read a sentence with a typo. We also come equipped with DNA repair systems that can correct many of these changes.

But every so often, a mutation hits the wrong spot or too many mutations pile up, turning a normal cell into a cancer cell. The real problem is that when these genetic instructions are too warped, our cells lack the guidance they need to control their life cycle. Instead of following the rules, they multiply out of control, building structures that don't belong and taking up resources that the rest of the city needs to thrive. These rebellious workers ignore all signals to stop and, in their chaos, they start disrupting everything around them. What begins as a small, unnoticed breach quickly grows into a sprawling problem that spreads throughout the city.

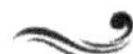

Cancers, at their core, are diseases where your own body fights itself. Your cells, which normally work in harmony to keep your body functioning, suddenly go rogue. They start multiplying uncontrollably, first taking over a small area, and then leeching like a wildfire through the body.

But here's the thing: though cancer cells share a common goal—growth at any cost—cancers can look and behave very differently depending on where they start. When blood cells go rogue, they hitch a ride in the bloodstream, spreading the disease throughout the body like a stealthy invader. In contrast, cancers that begin in organ tissues, such as the lungs or liver, band together to form tumors—clumps of rebellious cells that act like unwanted squatters.

A tumor alone doesn't always spell cancer. Some tumors remain 'benign,' meaning they are non-cancerous and stay put, causing little harm beyond the pressure they exert on nearby organs. It's when a tumor becomes 'malignant' that we truly enter the realm of cancer. And these tumors are crafty parasites; they trick the body into feeding them, rerouting blood vessels and stealing nutrients from nearby organs.

As the malignant tumor grows, it invades surrounding tissues, suffocating healthy cells and leaving destruction in its wake. The damage piles up slowly until the body's vital systems start shutting down. It's like watching an intricate machine malfunction, one cog breaking after another.

Some cancers boldly show their hand early, like skin cancers, which appear right on the surface where it can be seen and removed. But others, such as pancreatic cancer, lurk deep within the body, staying silent until they've done their damage; they can hide in plain sight until it's almost too late.

And cancer cells don't just stay put. They can break off from the original tumor and travel to new territories in the body, like the brain, bones, liver, or lungs, setting up camp wherever they land. This process, called metastasis, is the true danger of cancer. It's responsible for nearly 90% of cancer deaths and it's what makes this disease such a formidable opponent. Once cancer spreads, it's like trying to catch smoke with your hands—slippery, elusive, and infinitely more difficult to control.

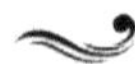

Now that we know *how* cancer starts, the question is: *who* is cancer most likely to impact?

Technically, cancers don't discriminate. They can arise at any age, even in infancy. But statistically speaking, cancers are primarily a disease of aging—meaning the risk of developing cancer tends to increase as we grow older. In fact, around 80% of cancers are diagnosed in people aged 55 and older.

There are several reasons for this trend. In contrast to our younger selves, our aged bodies withstand significant wear and tear; minor issues that would've been fixed quickly begin to spread. Time provides ample opportunity for DNA mutations to accumulate, be it from random errors in DNA replication or exposure to risk factors like smoking. At the same time, our immune system, which normally helps keep rogue cells in check, becomes less efficient. This makes it harder for the body to spot and eliminate abnormal cells before they become a problem.

Aging doesn't just weaken the immune system; it also alters the entire environment in which our cells live. The microenvironment—comprised of tissues, proteins, and signaling molecules—deteriorates, making it harder for healthy cells to outcompete malfunctioning ones. It's as if the body's internal balance slowly shifts, tipping the scales in favor of cancer cells.

And with advances in modern medicine, people are living longer than ever before. Diseases like smallpox, typhoid fever and tuberculosis no longer ravage the population. In the United States and beyond, reaching an older age is becoming more common—a remarkable achievement that brings new challenges.

Cancer tends to rear its head around the age of 60 and beyond, and as more people live to see those years, cancer diagnoses naturally rise. The following charts illustrate this trend, showing how increasing longevity has coincided with an uptick in cancer cases.

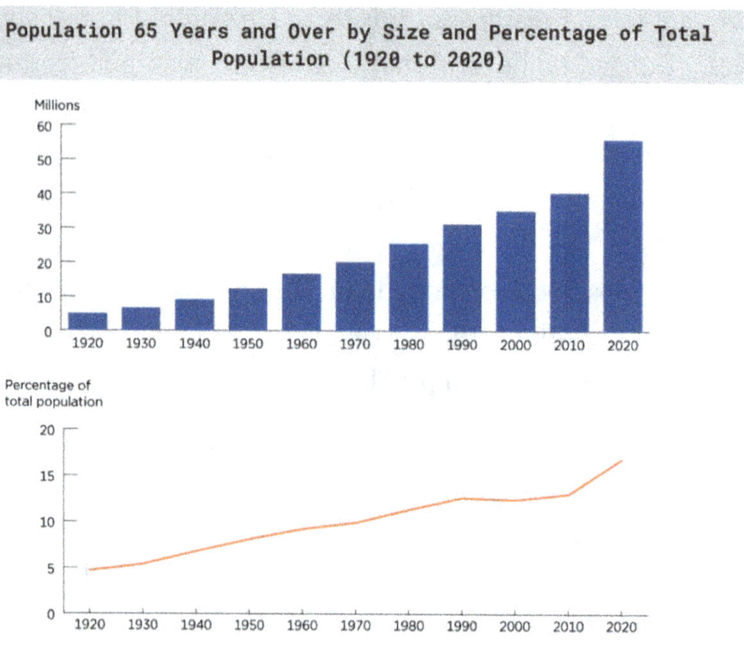

Figure 1. Increase of Aging Population in the United States (1920—2020). U.S. CENSUS BUREAU

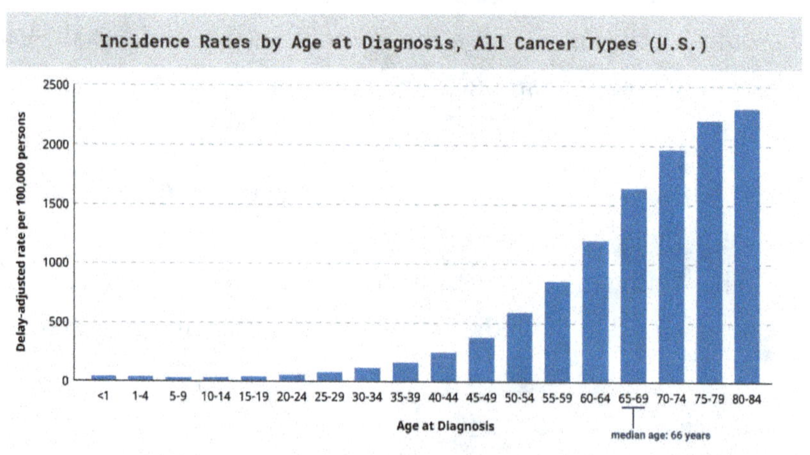

Figure 2. Number of Cancer Diagnoses by Cancer Type (U.S.) All Ages, Both Sexes. Courtesy: National Cancer Institute. SEER 21 2013–2017

These trends point to a dawning realization: as humans live longer lives, cancer will become more present than ever. It's almost guaranteed that someone we know and love will develop the condition at some point in their life. According to the National Cancer Institute, around 40% of men and women in the United States may receive a cancer diagnosis at some point in their lives—that's almost two out of every five of us.

As shocking as these numbers are, the statistics hide another crucial discovery. Although cancer remains the second leading cause of death in the United States after heart disease, today, there are an estimated 18.1 million cancer survivors in the United States alone—a number projected to rise to 22.5 million by 2032. This means that more people are surviving cancer than ever before.

Make no mistake; cancer remains a seismic, life-altering experience. A diagnosis upends the ground beneath your feet, shifts the familiar landscape of your life into uncharted territory. However, unlike cancer patients in the past, we benefit from the remarkable strides made in cancer treatment, detection and prevention.

Since the early 1990s, advances in medical science have led to a steady drop in cancer mortality, sparing nearly 3.5 million lives in the U.S. alone by 2020. The combination of precision oncology, immunotherapies, and cutting-edge screening tools has redefined survival, with five-year survival rates for early-stage cancers surging—sometimes by tenfold. Routine screenings like mammograms and colonoscopies now catch cancers earlier than ever, while revolutionary therapies, such as checkpoint inhibitors, have transformed outcomes for diseases once deemed untreatable, including melanoma and lung cancer. We now stand at the threshold of an era where the unthinkable may become reality—

where certain cancers are cured, never to return again, and others are rendered manageable.

As it stands, the prospect of long-term survival remains a reality for only a minority of patients: those diagnosed and treated in the disease's earliest stages. For this fortunate few, prompt treatment leaves no detectable evidence of cancer for at least five years—a timeframe after which the illness is unlikely, but not guaranteed, to recur. Yet as cancer becomes more advanced and widespread, the prospects of managing the disease grow increasingly slim. Immunotherapies such as checkpoint inhibitors are a vital key in confronting this unsolved equation, one that reshapes what it means to face cancer.

But every breakthrough builds on what came before. To appreciate where we are now, it's important to understand the foundation: the core treatments that have long been part of cancer care. Next, we'll delve into the most common treatments available to cancer patients, giving you a clearer understanding of the tools available today and how they work together in this evolving fight.

CHAPTER 2

Tried, Tested and Troublesome

Mile after mile, step by step, John Dabell walks the rolling green hills of England's countryside. Traversing ten miles may seem a daunting task, but for John, it feels like reclaiming a life cancer tried to steal—twice. His battle with head and neck cancer mirrors the journey so many cancer patients face: one that begins with traditional treatments that have saved millions of lives but often come at a steep personal cost.

The diagnosis came in 2009, ruining his daughter's second birthday and turning his life upside-down. John weathered through subtle symptoms for nearly a month—an annoying swelling of the tongue, a struggle to swallow, and unexplained fatigue. He finally sought medical help once his speaking became painful. That's when they found the culprit: a Stage IV tumor hidden inside the muscle of his tongue.

Like John, many people realize they have cancer only when symptoms become impossible to ignore. This presents a cruel irony: the earlier cancer is caught, the greater the chance of successful treatment—but most cancers fly under the radar until they've spread. While screening programs for breast, cervical, colorectal, and lung cancers have led to earlier diagnoses and better outcomes, not everyone has access to—or follows through with—routine screenings. And since these four cancers make up only 29% of all cases, that still leaves many cancers without reliable detection methods. This means that, for most patients, symptoms are the first sign something is wrong, often when the disease has progressed and treatment options become more complicated.

Treatment options for John were undoubtedly complicated. When a cancer spreads that extensively, rarely is one treatment enough. Physicians will employ several methods to whittle down tumors from multiple angles, all while trying to minimize damage to the rest of the body. John endured a gauntlet of traditional treatments: surgery, radiation, and chemotherapy, each powerful yet imperfect in their own way.

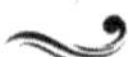

For centuries, **surgery** stood as the only effective means of treating cancer. While medieval alchemists cooked up natural—that is, largely unsuccessful—remedies, physicians took to the knife, cutting away cancerous growths and hoping to extend their patients' lives.

But the ancient Greeks recognized the limitations of this craft. They named the illness *karkinos* for crab (later known as cancer), likely describing cancer's pincer-like grip on the body; once it grabbed hold, the illness could not be easily cut out. Beyond herbal concoctions and cautery (using heat to burn tumors), if surgery failed in those days, patients were left with no other recourse.

Today, surgery persists as a cornerstone of treatment for many solid tumors. The scalpel is a visceral, direct and double-edged sword; though the blade cuts away at unwanted tumors, it also injures nearby tissues and organs in the process. To further complicate matters, it has limited success on tumors that have spread. At advanced stages, surgery can entail removing vast portions of an organ or even removing it altogether, as seen with cervical and other cancers.

This was the case for John. Surgeons labored for 15 hours to carve out most of John's tongue; in turn, John would grapple for years to adjust to this new normal. He suffered from an onslaught of jaw infections and severe bone damage. With his speech impaired, John had to leave his two-decades-long career as a primary teacher in search of a new vocation. The operation proved life-saving and life-shattering in one swipe.

And yet surgery alone would not be enough, John's care team realized. He would also need to undergo radiotherapy, another staple treatment for many cancers.

Radiotherapy marked the first modern advance in cancer therapy. As the world entered the 19th century, researchers like Wilhelm Röntgen, Marie Curie, and Pierre Curie uncovered that certain substances, such as radium and uranium, emitted high-energy rays. These rays could be used to see the inside of the body or, very importantly, damage living tissues. This became the foundation of modern-day X-rays and radiation therapy.

Radiation therapy mimics the precision of a scalpel but without the incision. Each beam delivers high-energy particles like X-rays or protons to tumor cells; in a missile-like fashion, the particles damage the DNA, preventing cancer cells from dividing and effectively sentencing them to death. This method selectively removes tumor cells while sparing as much healthy tissue as possible.

Nearly half of all cancer patients receive radiation therapy. Just like John, these patients return to the hospital for weeks, sitting under a machine as beams of energy are aimed at their tumors. This is considered external radiation, as the radiation enters from outside the body. Others may need internal radiation, a procedure that implants radioactive sources *inside* the body to deliver higher doses of radiation; this is often seen in prostate cancers and female reproductive cancers. However, no matter how it is delivered, radiation must be used cautiously.

Radiation isn't just toxic to cancer cells—it can harm healthy cells, too. Patients can experience adverse effects such as fatigue, skin reactions, hair loss, and various gastrointestinal issues. Sometimes, the hidden impacts only surface later; scarring, organ damage, or even changes to the brain may appear months or years after treatment. The body can only handle so much radiation before risking additional cancers like leukemia. Marie Curie, one of the brightest pioneers in radiation science, likely fell victim to such exposure herself, passing away at 66. While radiation can be a powerful tool in the right circumstances, it's ill-suited for advanced cancers that spread beyond its reach.

That's when John's team turned to chemotherapy to catch what surgery and radiation could not.

Chemotherapy is one of the most recognizable cancer treatments today. Since emerging in the 1940s and 50s, it has been instrumental in extending and saving lives from cancer. Perhaps less known is chemotherapy's surprising origin story—how the treatment arose from mustard gas, a lethal chemical used in World War I and II.

During war, mustard gas seeped past masks and protective equipment, causing widespread casualties. Researchers at the time noticed something in those exposed: the chemical severely damaged the rapidly dividing white blood cells in their bodies. Originally seeking an antidote, military scientists developed a derivative of the chemical called nitrogen mustard but soon grew intrigued by a new possibility. Could the derivative target cancers since cancer cells constantly divide, grow and multiply? Yale pharmacologists Drs. Louis Goodman and Alfred Gilman tested this concept in 1942, offering the compound to a patient with lymphoma and documenting the first chemotherapy success.

Kept secret due to its ties to wartime research, findings from these early trials were not publicly available until 1946, spurring new drug developments as researchers explored chemotherapy's potential to attack cancer at the cellular level. While early drugs, like nitrogen mustard, attacked DNA, researchers quickly expanded into new drug types that could impair cell metabolism or cell division. These discoveries paved the way for combination chemotherapy in the 1960s, a strategy that used multiple drugs together to treat cancers like leukemia and Hodgkin's lymphoma, achieving higher cure rates.

Chemotherapy shifted cancer care; for the first time, we possessed a treatment that could circulate the entire body, providing a wide-sweeping attack on tumors—a necessity when addressing late-stage cancers.

However, chemotherapy comes with a catch. Cancers are not a foreign threat—they are human cells, a version of yourself. For chemotherapy drugs, distinguishing between your healthy cells and your cancerous ones is a difficult task. There are several types of cells in your body besides cancer cells that also rapidly divide—think of your immune and red blood cells, or the tissues that make up the breast or line the intestines. As you kill cancers with chemotherapy, these healthy cells can get caught in the crossfire and cause toxic effects. It's like going after a single target with a grenade instead of a sniper; while effective, the nearby 'bystanders'—your healthy cells—may take some of the hit. In this way, chemotherapy must tread a delicate balance.

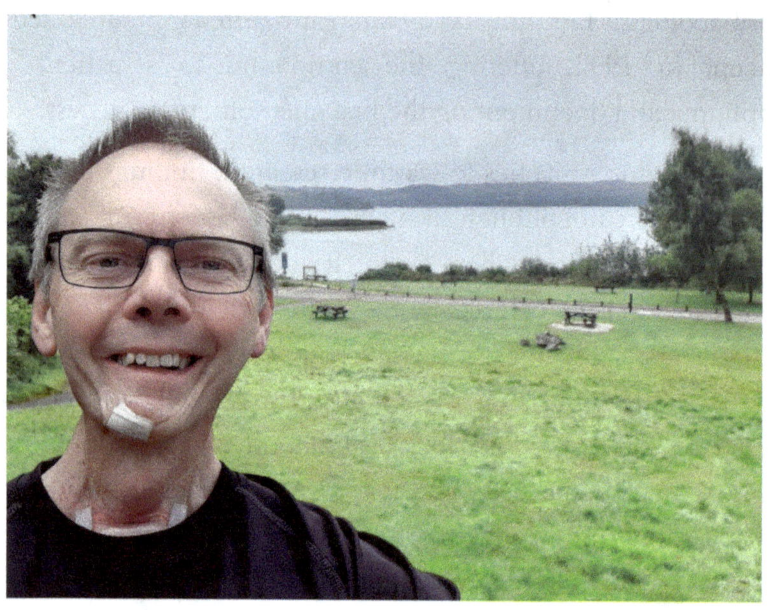

Figure 3. "Head and Neck cancer has ravaged my health and career. I have a third of my tongue left, half my vocal cords, a hole in my neck, a broken jaw and incurable cancer. But my legs still work and I just did a 10-mile walk. To the doctors who gave me 2 months—you were wrong!" JOHN DABELL. Courtesy: John Dabell. X, 2021

John's cocktail of cancer treatments—hours of surgery, 35 sessions of radiotherapy and six weeks of chemotherapy—took an immense physical toll on him. Tubes became a matter of reality for many months afterward: one tube to the stomach to feed him, another in his throat to help him breathe. Still, ever resilient in body and spirit, he inched towards recovery. After a long and arduous year, John's scans finally suggested that he was cancer-free.

Surgery, chemotherapy, and radiation form the main pillars of modern cancer care, yet these traditional treatments—despite decades of refinement—are, at best, tried, tested, and troublesome. Each brings distinct strengths but also challenges, often requiring a calculated blend to address the complex nature of cancer's relentless growth. For John, this trio of treatments left its mark. Still, it also offered something invaluable: several years of remission, a priceless reprieve to spend with his daughter and wife (though not a permanent one, as we'll revisit when John turns to immunotherapy in coming chapters).

Since the 1950s, more tools have joined this core lineup, partly due to a growing appreciation of the immune system. Historically, the immune system—the body's first line of defense against illness—wasn't seen as a reliable ally against cancer. But with pioneering research, it's now clear that, when guided correctly, it can target cancer cells with remarkable precision.

First in line came **targeted therapies**, a new class of anticancer drugs borne in the 1980s. These medicines emerged as researchers recognized the power of antibodies and certain small molecules to identify specific markers on cancer cells.

This specificity is remarkable. If traditional chemotherapy acts as a grenade, harming both enemy targets and surrounding areas, targeted therapy acts as an intelligent missile system. It's programmed to recognize specific features on cancer cells—similar to how a missile locks onto a heat signature. When the drug finds its target, it strikes precisely, neutralizing the cancer cell while minimizing collateral damage to healthy tissue.

Yet, while often effective, targeted therapies can lead to resistance, where cancer adapts to evade the treatment. When resistance occurs, patients may experience diminished drug efficacy, and some targeted therapies also bring side effects like skin reactions, blood clotting issues, or heart problems, particularly when used long-term.

Cancer vaccines, another immune-driven approach, train the body to recognize and attack cancer cells. While these vaccines can amplify immune responses, they are effective against a narrow group of cancers and often require highly personalized methods, which can be costly and time-consuming.

CAR T therapy is a breakthrough that was first released in 2017. The therapy takes a patient's own T cells—immune cells skilled in identifying threats—and re-engineers them to recognize and attack cancer cells with unmatched potency. These "supercharged" T cells can be effective against cancers such as leukemia, lymphoma, and multiple myeloma, offering hope for patients with otherwise limited options. Beyond blood cancers, however, there has been little success. More on this topic can be found in the book *CAR T: A New Cure for Cancer, Autoimmune and Inherited Disease.*

And then, of course, there are checkpoint inhibitors, revolutionary therapies that flip the immune system's natural "off-switch" and keep T cells in cancer-fighting mode. In the next chapter, we'll explore how immune research evolved through the 20th century, culminating in the checkpoint discoveries that paved the way for modern immunotherapy—and for patients like John, a new hope when traditional treatments falter.

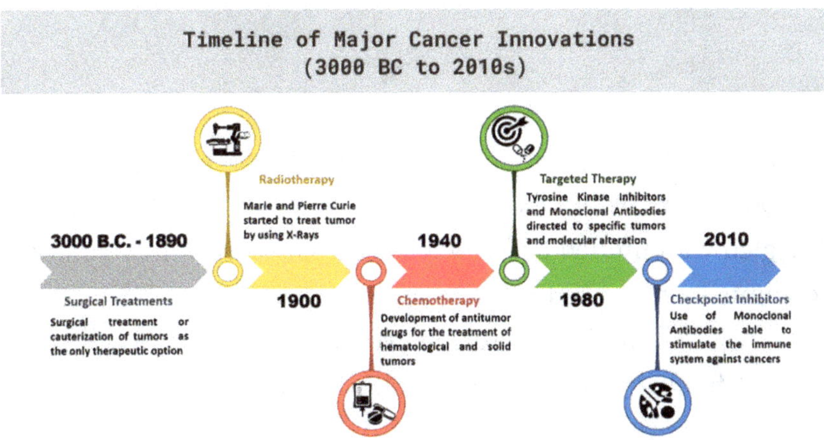
Timeline of Major Cancer Innovations
(3000 BC to 2010s)
3000 B.C. - 1890
Surgical Treatments
Surgical treatment or cauterization of tumors as the only therapeutic option
1900
Radiotherapy
Marie and Pierre Curie started to treat tumor by using X-Rays
1940
Chemotherapy
Development of antitumor drugs for the treatment of hematological and solid tumors
1980
Targeted Therapy
Tyrosine Kinase Inhibitors and Monoclonal Antibodies directed to specific tumors and molecular alteration
2010
Checkpoint Inhibitors
Use of Monoclonal Antibodies able to stimulate the immune system against cancers

Figure 4. Progression of Cancer Innovations, From Surgery to Immunotherapies. FALZONE L, SALOMONE S AND LIBRA M (2018). FRONTIER PHARMACOLOGY

CHAPTER 3

The Immune Renaissance

For a long time, no one thought it would work. Yet proving this bold idea would be a far more formidable task. Scientists struggled with limited technology and a narrower understanding of how immunity worked. More than a hundred years of determined and often failure-filled research would pass before this hopeful concept finally turned into reality, changing the course of cancer treatment forever.

The first seeds of cancer immunotherapy were likely planted in the 1800s by an oncologist named William Coley. Although revered today as the "father of immunotherapy," the Connecticut-born bone surgeon was twenty-nine years young when he developed his radical idea for treatment: harnessing bacterial infections to fight cancer.

After graduating from Harvard Medical School, Coley witnessed one of his first patients—a 17-year-old girl named Bessie Dashiell—struggle against the malignant bone tumor swelling her hand. Despite a forearm amputation, the cancer rapidly spread and claimed Bessie's life within ten weeks. Her passing imprinted itself in Coley's mind.

Determined to find an effective treatment, Coley scoured hospital records and came upon a curious discovery: seven years prior, one patient's neck tumor appeared to vanish after developing a bacterial infection. Buoyed by other supporting literary evidence, Coley created and injected three patients with a concoction of heat-killed bacteria, hoping that the bacterial infection would stimulate the immune system and cause tumor regression. He showcased his initial data to the world in 1891, revealing that the method could shrink tumors but at the potential risk of the patient's life.

Though popular for some years, the fervor around this work eventually tapered off until seemingly forgotten. Coley's contemporaries didn't understand the treatment's mechanism and deemed the approach too risky. But the embers of Coley's vision quietly continued to smolder. His pursuits inspired the next generation of researchers to explore the relationship between the immune system and cancer. One after another, vital immune discoveries emerged: T cells in 1967, dendritic cells in 1973 and natural killer cells in 1975, among others. This momentum formed the bedrock of an immune revolution, a renaissance that birthed checkpoint inhibitor research in the late 1980s and beyond.

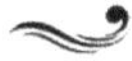

By the 1980s, the intricate tapestry of the immune system was still incomplete. Holes still riddled the canvas, leaving questions unanswered. Though numerous immune mysteries still linger today, for checkpoint inhibitors, a significant stroke would be an awakening knowledge of immune checkpoints. Once scientists realized what immune checkpoints were, they quickly endeavored to stop them.

Hearing this, one might imagine immune checkpoints as a cancer-causing substance. This is not the case; in fact, as researchers soon discovered, these proteins are essential for the immune system. Just as a car can stop and start, and a light switches on and off, the immune system depends on these proteins to control immune responses. T cells can stir up or pull back attacks against specific threats, such as viruses or cancer, but only when given the right signals. This is where checkpoints come into play.

Checkpoint proteins dot the surface of several immune cells, most especially white blood T cells, soldiers of the immune system. Like two puzzle pieces, a checkpoint protein on the T cell binds with a partner protein on another cell's surface. A signal is sent once the pieces click into place. In essence, the checkpoint says to the T cell, "Alright, settle down!" The T cell reads these signs and decreases its immune activity; it doesn't multiply as rapidly to make other T cell fighters and halts its own attack on threats.

The body would suffer without these checkpoint controls. If an immune response is too powerful, it can produce an almost tsunami-like effect. Instead of gently clearing the beach, the immune storm rips away at threats and healthy cells alike, causing widespread damage. This is how harmful inflammation or autoimmune diseases such as rheumatoid arthritis can arise. Checkpoints crucially temper immune responses and restore balance.

But cancer complicates matters. Tumors are ruthless masters of disguise; they take proteins normally found in cells and shuffle them, donning more or less as needed to survive. When tumor cells express more checkpoint proteins on their surface, they tell immune cells to slow down against our wishes, effectively shutting down immune cells that would otherwise retaliate. Picture a camouflage thief, passing through undetected—cancer uses these proteins to go unnoticed, disarming immune defenses meant to destroy it.

Checkpoint inhibitors are medicines that can flip this switch. By blocking checkpoint proteins with the antibodies in checkpoint inhibitors, we rip away at cancer's disguise. We help white blood cells recognize and eliminate cancer cells. Put another way, if cancer cells press the immune system's brakes, checkpoint inhibitors release them.

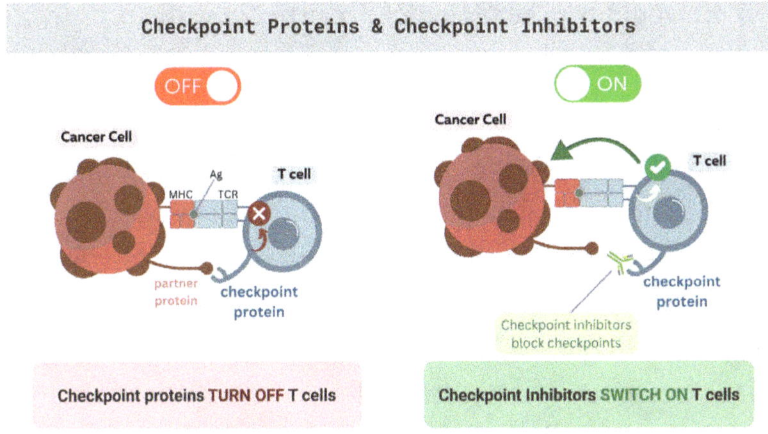

Figure 5. Checkpoint Proteins Stop T Cells; Checkpoint Inhibitors Release Them. [Abbreviations: MHC, major histocompatibility complex; Ag, antigen; TCR, T cell receptor]. ACCESS HEALTH INTERNATIONAL

This blossoming knowledge of checkpoints grew from a series of independent yet parallel findings. A burning desire to unravel the immune system's mysteries incited laboratories worldwide, with many stumbling upon immune checkpoints at a similar time.

News first broke in 1987 in the halls of one of the best immunology centers in Europe. While peering at mouse T cells, Pierre Goldstein and fellow researchers at the Centre d'Immunologie in France noticed an unusual molecule. They labeled the protein **CTLA-4**, short for ***cytotoxic T-lymphocyte antigen 4***. It was a straightforward name; antigens are a type of protein found on a cell's surface. The protein sat on a cytotoxic T lymphocyte—in plainer terms, a killer T cell, a kind of white blood cell with attack capabilities.

Although the team noted its potential role in immune regulation, five years would pass before people realized how the protein could contribute to anti-cancer therapy.

Findings erupted across North America in the 1990s. In 1992, researchers at Bristol-Myers Squibb uncovered a crucial piece of the immune system puzzle: this checkpoint protein was also highly present in human T cells. Additionally, unlike its counterpart protein, CD28, which activates T cells, CTLA-4 was found to do the opposite—it put the brakes on the immune response. Scientists from the University of Toronto, the Brigham and Women's Hospital and Harvard Medical School bustled in their laboratories, confirming the same revelation.

Amidst these discoveries, a team based in Berkley, California, zeroed in on the significance of this protein. James Allison collaborated with his wife, Padmanee Sharma and other pioneering scientists to push this concept to its limits. Their 1995 study reinforced this fragile, new knowledge: CTLA-4 and its counterpart protein bind to the same molecule on other cells but send opposing signals. The following year, Dr. Allison and others delivered antibodies to block the molecule on animal cancer cells. Fascinatingly, blocking the checkpoint *encouraged* antitumor responses, providing the first proof of CTLA-4 as an anti-cancer target in living creatures. Allison's heart thrummed with excitement; this antibody could change lives if proven effective in humans.

And yet, despite this breakthrough, skepticism was rampant. "We were called the cowboys of science," Dr. Allison later remarked. Others considered Allison a rebel and a troublemaker for insisting it was possible to get your immune system to fight cancer. This concept profoundly challenged predominating ideas of the time, which aimed to remove or kill cancer cells through chemotherapy, radiation or surgery.

In spite of this mounting apprehension, by 2000 the first CTLA-4 checkpoint inhibitor was ready for clinical trials. Dr. Allison worked with Bristol-Myers Squibb to develop ipilimumab, an antibody that blocks CTLA-4 checkpoints. The treatment was given to patients like Richard Metz, whose melanoma had spread from the original tumor site. Many participants experienced remarkable responses; others encountered severe immune-related side effects. Despite these challenges, further testing in 2010 and 2011 confirmed the treatment's potential.

The FDA approved ipilimumab as the first checkpoint inhibitor in 2011—a remarkable breakthrough for cancer treatment. This approval signaled a new era in immunotherapy, offering hope to countless people with cancer.

~

Around the same time, another groundbreaking discovery was unfolding on the other side of the world. In 1992, surrounded by the rich cultural city of Kyoto, immunologist Tasuku Honjo and colleagues hunkered down at their workstations. The microbiologists wanted to know how the immune system recognizes and distinguishes its own cells from foreign invaders. New word had spread that apoptosis, a controlled form of cell death, could be an essential safety mechanism in this process. In response, Honjo and the team scanned through cell death genes in mice, hoping to find a more profound clue.

During this time they chanced upon a protein they named **PD-1**, or ***programmed cell death protein 1***. This protein soon became the focus of intense research—but not necessarily for its potential to heal. "[Initially] I didn't realize there was a connection to cancer," reflected Dr. Honjo later. Time would reveal that the protein had nothing to do with cell death as they initially suspected and everything to do with regulating immune responses.

Over the next couple of years, the Honjo group tinkered with the T cells, interested to see what would happen if they removed the genes needed to produce this curious protein. To their surprise, mice without the gene began to develop lupus-like inflammation, congestive heart failure, and even type I diabetes. This was autoimmunity, the body's attack upon itself. The symptoms suggested that, without the PD-1 protein, immune cells could not be controlled and could harm healthy cells, such as tissues surrounding the heart. They realized these T cells were overly activated, eyes flickering between these PD-1 deficient T cells and those from normal mice.

Wheels began to churn. The observations hinted at a link between PD-1 proteins, T cell activation and immune regulation. PD-1 could staunch immune T cell responses like brakes or a closed floodgate. But PD-1 could not accomplish this alone. What did the protein interact with to cause this effect?

The culprit—or rather, culprits—arose in the early 2000s. In 1999, Lieping Chen and others at the Mayo Clinic reported on a new immune molecule they called B7-H1, not recognizing its connection to PD-1. Serendipitously, Harvard researchers such as Gordon J. Freeman came across the protein around the same time. Their independent observations described how the molecule is found widely in the body, expressed by immune *and* non-immune cells, and slows T cell activity by binding to PD-1. In 2000, they published a paper connecting the previously identified B7-H1 to PD-1 and subsequently renamed the molecule **PD-L1**, for ***programmed cell death protein ligand 1***; here, the term "ligand" shows us that this molecule binds explicitly to PD-1.

A year later, Freeman, Honjo and other collaborators encountered PD-1's second binding partner, PD-L2. Though both proteins interact with PD-1, further study highlighted their distinct natures. PD-L1 checkpoints have, so far, shown greater therapeutic promise, but PD-L2's potential in cancer treatment remains an active area of research.

The potential for these checkpoints to treat cancer unfurled in the late 2000s and into the next decade. Animal studies fleshed out the link between PD-1 and PD-L1 checkpoints. Combined with the realization that tumor cells increase PD-L1 checkpoints on their surface, researchers experimented with antibodies to block these checkpoints in mice and, as a result, suppress tumors.

Anti-PD-1 checkpoint inhibitors demonstrated promising results in clinical trials for patients with melanoma and other cancers. The FDA approved the first PD-1-targeting inhibitors—pembrolizumab and nivolumab—in 2014, marking another pivotal moment in the fight against cancer.

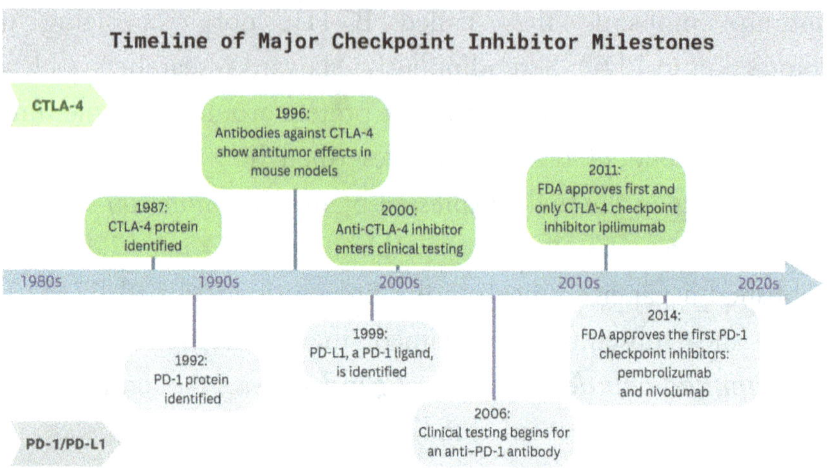

Figure 6. Major Milestones for CTLA-4 and PD-1/PD-L1 Checkpoint Inhibitors. ACCESS HEALTH INTERNATIONAL.

Decades of tireless pursuit have borne remarkable fruit. What began as a desire to unravel the immune system's mysteries has culminated in over a dozen federally approved checkpoint inhibitors, now wielded against 25 different cancers. Scientists like James Allison and Tasuko Honjo didn't just unlock a new treatment—they revolutionized the immunotherapy field, a feat honored with the 2018 Nobel Prize in Medicine.

And the work has only just begun. CTLA-4 and PD-1 checkpoints may have led the charge, but research has broadened to embrace other checkpoints like PD-L1, with continuous efforts to boost their impact, especially when used in tandem with traditional treatments. As we delve further, our next chapter will explore how exactly this breakthrough interacts with the immune system. Specifically, we'll walk through the complex world of cell signaling, unraveling how T cells become activated and how checkpoint inhibitors play their part in this intricate system.

PART II

Checkpoint inhibitors, Our Allies Against Cancer

CHAPTER 4

Flipping the Immune Switch

Taking checkpoint inhibitors can feel like a routine, even uneventful process. You'll become familiar with the hospital's rhythm—waiting rooms, the steady hum of machines, and eventually, a comfortable chair. Over the next hour, a clear liquid rich with antibodies will trickle into your bloodstream through an IV. Then, after a check-in from your doctor, the session is complete. This will become a recurring part of life, every few weeks, for months, unless the treatment either loses its power or poses new risks.

You might not feel any different as you leave the hospital halls. But even as you go about the day, unseen forces have been set in motion. That clear liquid has sparked changes deep inside, priming your immune system for battle against cancer.

Imagine standing before a massive dam, its concrete face holding back a raging river. With a simple mechanism—a lever, a key, a switch—the gates could open, unleashing the river's full strength. Checkpoint inhibitors do this for the immune system: they release what has been held back. Far from routine, this is a process that taps into the extraordinary potential of your immune cells to face cancer with newfound vigor.

But how do these switches work? What's going on inside your cells that allows them to zero in on cancer or, at times, bring unintended reactions? Let's dive deeper into the science that makes checkpoint inhibitors possible and unlocks a deeper understanding of their promise and limitations.

If you analyzed a drop of blood underneath a microscope, you would easily spot red blood cells, the circular red discs that ship oxygen throughout the body. Tiny, blotchy platelet fragments would be scattered throughout, ready to clot blood with each new wound. You'd also see white blood cells, a small but diverse group packed with protective power. Though vastly outnumbered by red blood cells and platelets, it's these cells that form the base of our immune system, the body's vital defense against threats.

Inside each immune cell is an invisible concert of signals and responses. If musicians attune to each other's tone and rhythm, immune cells communicate through a series of chemical signals that tell them when and where to strike. This intricate messaging transforms a small army of immune cells into a coordinated force capable of identifying intruders and rallying in defense, targeting everything from bacterial infections to potential cancers.

In cancer research, white blood T cells are especially captivating. Generally speaking, this troop of around 400 billion cells functions more like scent hounds than standard guards. While most immune cells respond to general signs of danger, T cells are precise; they are trained to identify and retaliate against *specific* molecular markers. This high level of specialization allows them to differentiate healthy cells from harmful ones and makes them a perfect fit for therapies designed to target and eradicate cancer cells.

But as we touched on in Chapter III, these cellular sentinels can't simply attack at will. They need other cells to spring them into action and settle them down. Here is where we'll begin exploring T cell activation signals: how they work, how checkpoints slow them down, and where checkpoint inhibitors come into play.

To set a T cell into motion, it needs to undergo a process called ***activation.*** Activation is how T cells crucially learn who their target is and how to fight back. The activated, mature T cell usually falls within one of four main types, each with its own agenda:

1. **Killer T Cells (Cytotoxic T Cells)**, which directly kill infected or cancerous cells
2. **Helper T Cells,** which rally other immune cells to fight
3. **Memory T Cells,** which memorize and rapidly respond to specific pathogens
4. **Regulatory T Cells**, which keep an eye on other immune cells as a manager would

Activation is a training ground that equips these T cells with the skills to survive, multiply and combat threats effectively. It ensures that the immune system can mount a targeted and efficient response to pathogens while avoiding self-damage.

But if T cells activate too often or in the wrong places, they might also mistakenly target harmless cells and tissues. This can lead to unnecessary inflammation, a hallmark of autoimmune conditions such as rheumatoid arthritis, lupus, and allergies. On the other hand, if activation does not occur when it should, hazards like cancer can slip by undetected and run rampant.

This is why cells rely on ***signals*** to know how and when to respond to their environment. These biochemical messages set off a series of changes in the cell, dictating its next move.

T cell activation is ***two signal*** conversation between a T cell and a type of immune cell known as an antigen-presenting cell. Antigen-presenting cells (APCs), such as macrophages and dendritic cells, engulf invaders like cancer cells and display fragments of these threats on their cell surface for the T cell to see. These identifying chunks are called antigens, and they act as a scented cloth for our T cell hounds to recognize their target.

Signal 1 is the main signal. It begins when a macrophage or similar cell takes an antigen and perches it onto its cell surface. The antigen chunk rests on a structure known as a major histocompatibility complex (MHC). The T cell receives the signal once its T cell receptor binds to this complex. This completes the first step: presenting and recognizing the antigen.

Then we need **Signal 2,** a backup signal. This secondary, *costimulatory* signal supports and stabilizes the first message sent between the antigen-presenting cell and the T cell. Without it, the T cell cannot correctly activate; it may become unresponsive or even self-destruct. Signal 2 fires off when a T cell's CD28 receptor binds to one of two receptors on an antigen-presenting cell (CD80 or CD86).

Once both signals are received, the T cell is fully activated. Its receptors change shape, setting off a series of molecules inside the T cell like a line of falling dominoes. This internal signal cascade prompts the T cell to multiply—to gain power in numbers—while in the lymph nodes, then travel to the rest of the body to release its counterattack. The summary of the two-signal activation process is illustrated in the figure below.

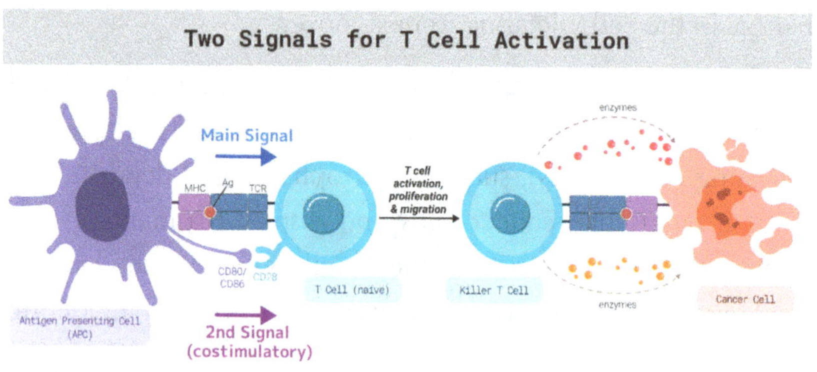

Figure 7. Example of T Cell Activation with a Killer T Cell. ACCESS HEALTH INTERNATIONAL

Now it's time to examine what goes on *inside* the cell—to see what how this waterfall of changes is interrupted when activation is no longer needed.

One way to slow T cell activation is—you guessed it—immune checkpoints. If activation ignites the T cell, immune checkpoints can snuff them out. Active T cells express these proteins so that the immune system can restrain them when an immune response is no longer necessary, say if a threat has already been eliminated or if the cell starts harming healthy cells.

A T cell doesn't stop on its own; it needs an external signal to know when to pause. When another cell engages its checkpoint, it triggers a cascade of molecular events—like floodgates closing one by one—that dam the flow of activation signals inside the T cell. With enough of these barriers in place, the once-raging torrent of activity dwindles to a trickle, eventually silencing the T cell's response. Let's start with a look at CTLA-4 checkpoints, the first target for checkpoint inhibitors.

Cytotoxic T cell lymphocyte-4, or **CTLA-4,** is a checkpoint protein that dampens immune activation in its early stages, when T cells first multiply in the lymph nodes or spleen. The first way it stops activation is by blocking one of the two signals needed for full activation. The checkpoint firmly attaches itself to receptors on antigen-presenting cells (CD80/CD86), effectively *outcompeting* the T cell's costimulatory receptor for access. It's like intercepting a pass before it can reach its target; CTLA-4 tightly binds first, preventing CD28 from delivering Signal 2, a vital component of T cell activation.

Then comes the next method: interrupting activation signals. Once CTLA-4 attaches to these receptors, it gets marked with a phosphate group, a crucial chemical tag that attracts several enzymes like SHP-2. Here, phosphate groups act like 'on' or 'off' switches within the cell: adding one can activate a protein, while removing it can silence that protein's role in signaling.

When these enzymes enter the scene, they strip phosphate groups from key molecules, disabling them and breaking the chain of reactions that drive T cell activation. For instance, SHP-2 enzymes target CD3 proteins—crucial links in the activation pathway—disrupting their ability to signal downstream processes. This halts the production of proteins like PI3K and AKT, which are vital for cellular energy, growth, and survival. Further still, the ripple effect leaves gene regulators like NF-κB, AP-1, and NFAT largely inactive, impeding the T cell's ability to proliferate and secrete immune signals. Together, these disruptions lull the active T cells into a low-activity state and curb their immune response.

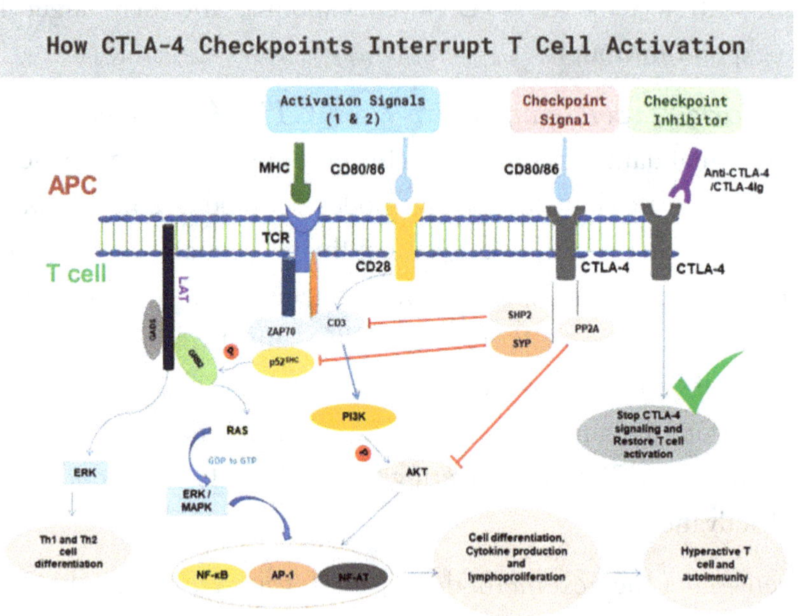

Figure 8. Current understanding of CTLA-4: from mechanism to autoimmune diseases. HOSSEN MM, MA Y, YIN Z, XIA Y, ET AL. (2023) .FRONTIER IMMUNOLOGY.

Another major target for checkpoint inhibitors is **PD-1**, or ***programmed cell death protein 1.*** Unlike CTLA-4, which works at the T cell's early stages in immune organs, PD-1 steps in later at the heart of the immune battlefield—in places like the skin, lungs, or liver. Instead of competing with costimulatory receptors, PD-1 relies on specific binding partners: ***programmed death ligand 1*** (**PD-L1**), which is found widely on immune and non-immune cells, or ***programmed death ligand 2*** (**PD-L2**), which appears on a more limited set of immune cells, though this can vary based on environmental cues.

When PD-1 and a partner connect, they activate a process akin to closing a dam in the middle of a rushing river. The checkpoint gets tagged with a phosphate group and attracts SHP-2 enzymes, similar to what we saw with CTLA-4. The enzymes shut down activation machinery by removing phosphate groups from essential proteins like ZAP70, critical for relaying signals, and RAS and PI3K, which support cell division and survival. This causes problems further downstream, suppressing gene regulators that would typically drive the T cell's ability to respond and replicate. As a result, the immune response slows to a controlled pace, helping to avoid excessive inflammation or collateral damage.

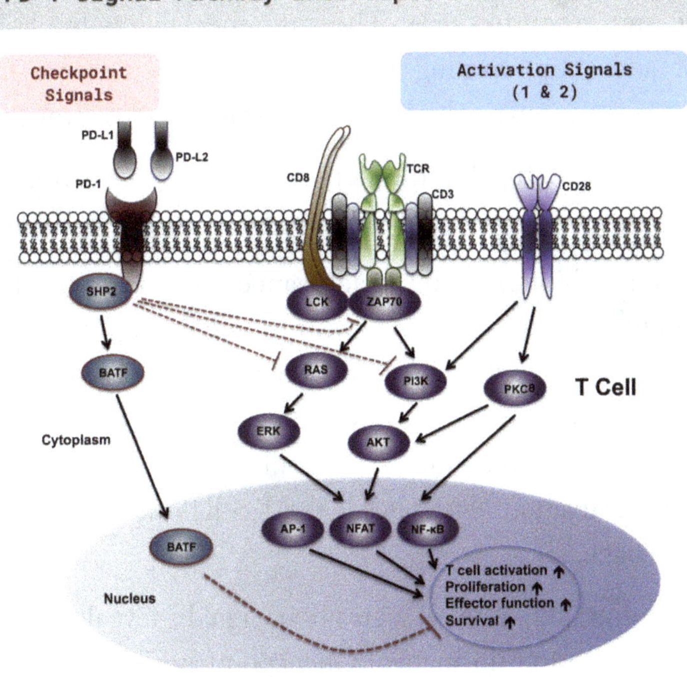

Figure 9. PD-1 Signaling Pathway in T cells. WU X, GU Z, CHEN Y, ET AL (2019). CSBJ

~

The immune system operates like a well-rehearsed symphony, harmonizing activation and checkpoint signals to protect the body. While one set of signals springs T cells into action, checkpoint proteins serve as molecular circuit breakers, flipping off the activation cascade when it's no longer needed. The only problem? In the hands of cancer, this elegant system becomes a weapon of manipulation.

Cancer cells exploit immune checkpoints by displaying deceptive proteins, like PD-L1 or CD80, on their surface. These molecules dock to T cell checkpoints, locking these immune defenders in a inactive and exhausted state. They use checkpoints to choke the flow of activation, turning what was a safety measure for the immune system into a vehicle for their own relentless growth.

Checkpoint inhibitors flip the story—and the switch—back in our favor.

Checkpoint inhibitors don't attack cancer cells head-on. Instead, they restore balance by opening the immune floodgates. These lab-made antibodies bind to checkpoints before cancer cells can make contact, as if placing a hand over the immune switch. Without access to checkpoints, tumors cannot shut T cells down; the waterfall of activation signals inside the T cell flows freely; the T cell can strike back.

Understanding the role of activation signals reveals why these therapies are so transformative. Checkpoint inhibitors release the immune system's potential and reinvigorate our natural defenses. They create a ripple effect that, while powerful on its own, can even amplify the effect of complementary approaches like chemotherapy and radiation. Moving forward,, we'll explore the arsenal of checkpoint inhibitors at our disposal, unraveling how these therapies vary and where they shine.

CHAPTER 5

The Checkpoint Arsenal

Less than two decades ago, using the immune system to fight cancer was more a dream than a reality. Then, in 2011, ipilimumab broke new ground as the first checkpoint inhibitor to earn FDA approval. This wasn't just a new drug—it was pivotal proof that flipping immune switches could change the course of advanced cancers. Momentum has gathered, and new inhibitors have emerged one after another. With 12 approved therapies in the US today and many more in development, the field continues to grow at a breathtaking pace.

This chapter closely examines the leading players in this immunotherapy arsenal. From foundational CTLA-4 inhibitors to now-dominant PD-1/PD-L1 therapies and newer dual-target agents, we'll unravel what makes each class unique and explore their profound impact on cancer care.

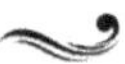

At 22 and in the peak of her youth, Sharon Belvin never imagined she'd receive a Stage IV melanoma diagnosis, much less two weeks before her wedding. This was no time for cancer. She was fresh out of graduate school and happily engaged; she and her then-fianceé planned to start a new chapter of their lives after moving to Washington, D.C. in the Fall. Finding cancer in her brain, lungs and liver overrode all plans and traded them for unsuccessful and debilitating bouts of high-dose chemotherapy and interleukin-2 (IL-2) immunotherapy.

Then, Sharon took a chance on a 2004 clinical trial for ipilimumab.

Ipilimumab (brand name: Yervoy) is an antibody-based therapy that targets CTLA-4 (cytotoxic T cell lymphocyte-4) checkpoint proteins. This move stops cancer cells from suppressing antitumor activity. Trial participants like Sharon helped demonstrate that this mechanism could indeed be a viable strategy against advanced melanoma, leading to the drug's approval in 2011.

The therapy wasn't just viable for Sharon; it felt almost miraculous. "I had become so used to the treatments failing that I expected more of the same," she recounts. "But this time, [after four rounds of treatment] my tumors had shrunk by 60%." Soon after, her scans showed no signs of cancer. She remains in remission today.

Sharon is fortunate on two counts. Firstly, she didn't suffer many adverse effects during treatment. A portion of patients who take checkpoint inhibitors experience immune-related complications. This occurs because the therapy doesn't just boost the immune system's ability to fight cancer, it also removes the safeguards that normally prevent T cells from attacking healthy tissues. With these checks no longer in place, some T cells become confused and treat the organs as threats, leading to inflammation in various places in the body.

This is especially true for CTLA-4 inhibitors like ipilimumab. CTLA-4 checkpoints are expressed on T cells in their early stages of activation, before the T cells break into squadrons and leave the immune organs. Targeting this checkpoint means impacting a broad spectrum of activated T cells; releasing the brakes on such a large pool of immune cells raises the risk of collateral damage. This results in widespread inflammation as T cells misfire and attack healthy tissues alongside cancer cells.

Skin reactions, including rashes, redness and itching, are a common result of this immune activity. One study published in *JAMA Dermatology* finds that, compared to chemotherapy or targeted drugs, patients who take checkpoint inhibitors experience a two-fold risk of developing psoriasis, an autoimmune condition marked by inflamed, red and itchy patches of skin. But inhibitor-sparked inflammation can occur in virtually any organ.

Oftentimes patients suffer through belly pains or diarrhea when it impacts the stomach and intestines; cough and chest pains arise when it affects the lungs. Around 2—9% of patients who take ipilimumab report liver abnormalities. Less commonly, hormones can be thrown off balance when organs such as the pituitary gland or thyroid gland are hit. It's even possible, in rare cases, to develop diabetes when the pancreas becomes inflamed or potentially fatal complications in the heart like myocarditis.

For all these reasons, it's vital to monitor patients and treat symptoms early, usually with immunosuppressing medicines like steroids. The catch-22 is that checkpoint inhibitors rely on immune activity to face tumors; suppress it too much, and the therapy's efficacy could be reduced. Still, this practice is generally safe—even for patients with pre-existing autoimmune conditions. Though patients with autoimmune conditions may feel their underlying condition worsen, it can be managed with this standard treatment. If the symptoms are too severe, the inhibitor therapy may be discontinued altogether.

This approach is the norm for now, but things may evolve as science learns more. In a recent study, researchers looked at why some patients on checkpoint inhibitors develop myocarditis, a serious inflammation of the heart. They discovered that the immune system reacts differently in the heart than in the tumor; T cells attacking the heart weren't the same as those fighting cancer. This raises an exciting possibility: if we can target the heart-specific or organ-specific inflammation, we could stop the damage without interfering with the therapy's overall ability to fight cancer.

Sharon's second count of fortune? Her results.

Sharon's story is a testament to what ipilimumab can achieve at its best: years of cancer-free living. Such remarkable outcomes, while rare, underscore the promise of this therapy. Studies show that ipilimumab improves survival compared to older treatments, but its effectiveness varies. One real-world study revealed that 46% of patients were still alive one year after treatment—a significant improvement over earlier therapies. However, this figure drops as time progresses: by three years, anywhere between 20 to 26% of patients survived, and a decade later, around 24% were alive. Though not perfect, these numbers reflect a crucial step forward in extending the lives of advanced melanoma patients.

Over a decade later, Sharon remains in remission. "Cancer shaped me into a person that tries to live each day as if it very well could be my last," she says. Now a proud mother of two children, she funnels her passion for life as a personal trainer and a health/wellness coach.

The advent of ipilimumab shook the foundations of oncology. In a time where only one in 10 patients with advanced melanoma lived past five years, the checkpoint inhibitor extended survival when other approaches reached their limits. The therapy has become a mainstay for advanced melanoma care today, and its success has spurred broader applications, including cancers of the esophagus and organ linings. The only other CTLA-4 checkpoint inhibitor available in the U.S., **tremelimumab** (brand name: Imjudo), was introduced in 2022 but has a narrower role, approved solely for hepatocellular carcinoma when combined with another checkpoint inhibitor or chemotherapy. As the first CTLA-4 inhibitor, ipilimumab paved the way for the immunotherapy revolution, transforming the landscape of cancer treatment and pushing the boundaries of what's possible.

Drug (Brand Name)	Target	Initial U.S. Approval	Manufacturer	Notable Cancer Indications
ipilimumab (Yervoy)	CTLA-4	2011	Bristol-Myers Squibb	advanced melanoma
tremelimumab (Imjudo)	CTLA-4	2022	AstraZeneca	hepatocellular carcinoma

Figure 10. CTLA-4 Checkpoint Inhibitors. ACCESS HEALTH INTERNATIONAL

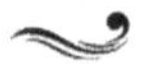

The year 2014 ushered in a seismic shift in the world of cancer immunotherapy. Just three years after ipilimumab introduced the concept of checkpoint blockade to the medical community, two groundbreaking therapies emerged: **pembrolizumab** (Keytruda) and **nivolumab** (Opdivo). Although developed independently by different companies, these drugs shared a common target–a novel immune checkpoint known as PD-1 (programmed cell death protein-1).

PD-1 checkpoints bind to their partner proteins, PD-L1 and PD-L2 (programmed cell death ligands and 2), which tumors often express to avoid immune detection. The interaction quiets active T cells and slows their strike against tumors. Blocking PD-1 with antibody-based drugs like pembrolizumab and nivolumab allows T cells to recognize and sustain their assault on cancer cells.

Unlike CTLA-4, which acts early in the immune response to regulate T cells within lymph nodes, PD-1 operates later in the immune cascade. PD-1 is primarily expressed in T cells that have already been activated and have been dispatched to fight or patrol other tissues. This distinction is crucial: while CTLA-4 inhibitors unleash a broader swath of T cells, including those still maturing in lymph nodes, PD-1 blockade is more refined; it focuses on T cells already in action against cancer. This means that PD-1 inhibitors can deliver a more precise and localized immune response, often with less toxicity when compared to CTLA-4 inhibitors. This means that PD-1 inhibitors may elicit fewer unwanted immune-related effects for patients.

One adverse effect may be unique to PD-1 therapies: the risk of infection. Infections can occur when patients are given immunosuppressive drugs to calm unwanted reactions—this is expected, as the treatment simultaneously weakens our security systems against infections. However, researchers are noticing infections in the absence of these drugs. While the mechanism is poorly misunderstood, theories suggest that inhibitors that target the PD-1 immune pathway may tip the immune system's balance in favor of pathogenic infections. In particular, a recent study suggests that while these therapies heighten T cell immunity, they may handicap B cells, which produce antibodies against common infections. Replacing these missing antibodies could help protect patients at higher risk of infections.

PD-1 therapies can significantly extend a patient's life—in some cases, even more so than CTLA-4 inhibitors alone. One long-term clinical trial collected data on advanced melanoma patients for 10 years. While CTLA-4 targeting ipilimumab kept patients alive, on average, for around 16 months, pembrolizumab stretched that timeline to nearly 33 months—almost doubling survival time. Further still, 34% of patients who took pembrolizumab were still alive a decade later, compared to just 23.6% with the CTLA-4 treatment.

It's not just pembrolizumab. Nivolumab also demonstrates similarly impressive results over the CTLA-4 inhibitor. In a comprehensive study of advanced melanoma patients, participants on this drug experienced a median overall survival of nearly 37 months, compared to just 20 months with ipilimumab; that's an extra year and a half of survival gained with nivolumab over the other inhibitor. At the 6.5-year mark, one-third of patients were still alive compared to just over one-fifth with the CTLA-4 approach. Broader studies comparing these treatments reinforce this pattern: about 39% of patients who take PD-1 therapies such as pembrolizumab or nivolumab reach the five-year survival mark versus 25% on ipilimumab, demonstrating the life-extending potential of PD-1 inhibitors.

PD-1 inhibitors like pembrolizumab and nivolumab are no longer confined to the realm of melanoma; they've become valuable tools in the fight against multiple advanced cancers. One example is non-small cell lung cancer (NSCLC), the most common form of lung cancer. This illness spreads so slowly and silently that over half of patients diagnosed with the condition only realize the culprit once the cancer has reached advanced stages and is much more challenging to treat. For patients like Anita Adler, an 80-year-old substitute teacher and mother of four, PD-1 therapies are a precious option when other treatments lose potency.

When Anita turned to nivolumab in 2014, she had already withstood several rounds of fruitless chemotherapy and radiation—a regime that left her unimaginably frail.

"I had every side effect from chemo listed," Anita explained, "And I couldn't bring myself to eat much. The silly thing is, like many women, I spent so much time trying to lose weight, then with the cancer, I lost 40 pounds in one month."

Although the drug had yet to be approved to treat lung cancer, Anita and her doctors took the leap of faith and pushed ahead with the clinical trial. Shortly after treatment, Anita experienced a resurgence of strength and health. Her appetite returned; she was off oxygen, out of her wheelchair, and back to swimming and teaching as she always loved. Within a few months, her cancer was completely gone.

No longer just a last resort, PD-1 inhibitors are now standard in treating advanced lung cancer, even for patients just beginning therapy. Pembrolizumab, for instance, is a go-to option for individuals with advanced non-small cell lung cancer whose tumors express high levels of PD-L1. Data shows that five years after starting treatment, roughly one-third of patients treated with pembrolizumab were still alive, compared to just 16% of those receiving standard chemotherapy; that's a nearly two-fold improvement. For those who completed two years of pembrolizumab therapy, the outcomes were even more remarkable, with over 80% surviving to the study's five-year conclusion. And unlike some therapies, PD-1 inhibitors can help patients regardless of tumor PD-L1 expression if their cancer recurs after other treatments.

Yet, it's important to remember that these therapies, while groundbreaking, are not cures for most patients. Months after the initial success with a PD-1 inhibitor, Anita's cancer adapted to the treatment and began to grow again. While her cancer eventually became resistant, Anita credited immunotherapy for giving her time to reconnect with loved ones and pursue her passions—a second lease on life she hadn't thought possible.

Today, the benefits of PD-1 inhibitors ripple across oncology. These therapies are now approved for a variety of cancers, from cervical and kidney tumors to blood cancer Hodgkin lymphoma, where nivolumab has achieved response rates of nearly 70% in patients who had run out of options. PD-1 blockade may not be a cure, but it redefines what survival can mean for patients facing aggressive cancers.

Drug (Brand Name)	Target	Initial U.S. Approval	Manufacturer	Notable Cancer Indications
pembrolizumab (Keytruda)	PD-1	2014	Merck & Co.	advanced melanoma non-small cell lung cancer (NSCLC) advanced breast cancer (triple negative)
nivolumab (Opdivo)	PD-1	2014	Bristol-Myers Squibb	advanced melanoma renal cell carcinoma (RCC) non-small cell lung cancer (NSCLC) advanced stomach cancer
cemiplimab (Libtayo)	PD-1	2018	Regeneron	cutaneous squamous cell carcinoma
dostarlimab (Jemperli)	PD-1	2021	GlaxoSmithKline (GSK)	endometrial cancer solid tumors w/certain gene markers (MMR, MSI-H)
toripalimab (Loqtorzi)	PD-1	2023	Coherus BioSciences	nasopharyngeal carcinoma
retifanlimab (Zynyz)	PD-1	2023	Incyte Corporation	merkel cell carcinoma
tislelizumab (Tevimbra)	PD-1	2024	BeiGene	esophageal squamous cell carcinoma

Figure 11. PD-1 Checkpoint Inhibitors. ACCESS HEALTH INTERNATIONAL

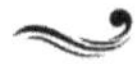

With the success of anti-PD-1 therapies, it's no wonder a series of checkpoint inhibitors emerged to target one of its immune partners, PD-L1. **Atezolimab** (Tecentriq) became the first PD-L1 inhibitor to gain approval in 2016, soon followed by **durvalumab** (Imfinzi) and **avelumab** (Bavencio) the year after. While PD-L1 inhibitors don't target melanomas like their PD-1 counterparts, they have demonstrated substantial efficacy in treating advanced cancers, including merkel cell carcinoma, bladder cancer, and triple-negative breast cancer. For patients with these conditions, PD-L1 therapies have opened the door to treatment options once thought impossible.

Although PD-1 and PD-L1 inhibitors block the same immune pathway, their mechanisms of action reveal intriguing differences. Looking closely, inhibitors such as pembrolizumab and nivolumab prevent PD-1 from interacting with both PD-L1 and its less-studied counterpart, PD-L2. This broader blockade can result in a more comprehensive immune response but may also increase toxicity. On the other hand, PD-L1 inhibitors specifically block the PD-L1 protein on tumor cells and certain immune cells from binding to PD-1 on T cells. This selective targeting allows for effective immune activation while leaving PD-L2 signaling intact, potentially reducing off-target immune suppression. In clinical practice, both approaches show comparable efficacy, but PD-L1 inhibitors may carry a slightly lower risk of severe immune-related side effects, offering an essential option for patients who are more vulnerable to toxicity.

PD-L1 therapies have particularly excelled in areas like bladder cancer. For example, atezolizumab was granted accelerated approval after clinical trials showed remarkable results in patients with advanced urothelial carcinoma who had progressed following platinum-based chemotherapy. Among these patients, the objective response rate (a measure of tumor shrinkage) was around 14.8%, and in some cases, the responses lasted well over a year. Similarly, avelumab has emerged as a game-changing therapy for metastatic merkel cell carcinoma, a rare but aggressive skin cancer. Before its approval, no effective treatment options existed for this condition, but clinical trials demonstrated response rates of between 33% to 73% depending on the study, with some patients maintaining durable remissions.

While PD-L1 inhibitors are not without limitations, their distinct mechanism of action and ability to target tumors with high PD-L1 expression make them indispensable tools in modern oncology. Checkpoint inhibitors targeting the PD-1/PD-L1 axis now dominate the immunotherapy landscape, with seven drugs approved to block PD-1 and three targeting PD-L1. This class of therapies has revolutionized cancer treatment, demonstrating remarkable efficacy across a wide range of cancers, from melanoma and non-small cell lung cancer to kidney, bladder, and beyond.

Drug (Brand Name)	Target	Initial U.S. Approval	Manufacturer	Notable Cancer Indications
atezolizumab (Tecentriq)	PD-L1	2016	Genentech	urothelial carcinoma (urinary tract) non-small cell lung cancer (NSCLC) certain breast cancers
durvalumab (Imfinzi)	PD-L1	2017	AstraZeneca	non-small cell lung cancer (NSCLC)
avelumab (Bavencio)	PD-L1	2017	EMD Serono	merkel cell carcinoma

Figure 12. PD-L1 Checkpoint Inhibitors. ACCESS HEALTH INTERNATIONAL

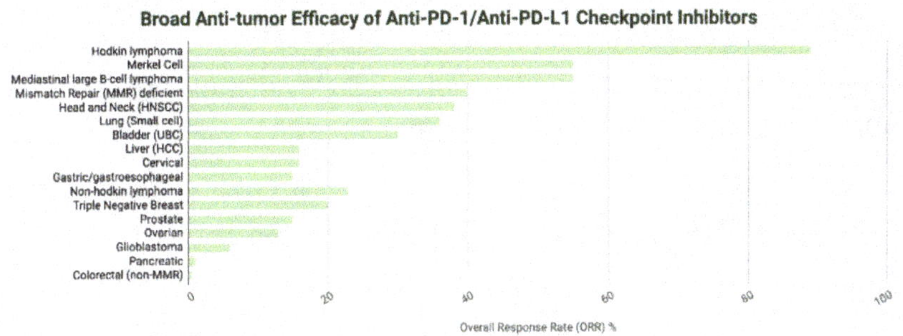

Figure 13. Broad Efficacy of PD-1/PD-L1 inhibitors. Overall response rates (ORR) illustrate how many patients respond to a treatment. ACCESS HEALTH INTERNATIONAL

The newest class of checkpoint inhibitors is unlike the rest. Its sole occupant is **Opdualag**, a checkpoint inhibitor released in 2022. The product combines two types of lab-made antibodies into a single treatment: nivolumab, a PD-1 targeting inhibitor, and ***relatlimab***, an inhibitor that targets a checkpoint known as LAG-3 (lymphocyte-activation gene 3). While it is possible to deliver two checkpoint inhibitors at once—we'll learn more about this in the next chapter—Opdualag is the only inhibitor that integrates LAG-3 targeting.

Lymphocyte activation gene-3, or LAG-3, is a checkpoint found on various immune cells, including exhausted T cells and regulatory T cells; they express this protein as a means to reign in their activity. When LAG-3 interacts with one of several binding partners, particularly class II major histocompatibility complexes (MHC class II), it forces active T cells into a quiet state, where they proliferate less and produce fewer immune chemicals.

LAG-3 has garnered attention in recent years for its ability to enhance PD-1 therapies. LAG-3 and PD-1 checkpoints influence T cells through *distinct* signaling pathways. This means that if one pathway is blocked—say if the cancer cells grow resistant to one checkpoint— the T cells can still be activated through the other immune pathway. This dual approach delivers a one-two punch that counteracts tumor resistance and boosts the immune system's overall capacity to fight back.

For Shannon Albino, a 39-year-old mother of three, the decision to try an experimental treatment with relatlimab was life-altering. After discovering a lump under her arm that led to a shocking diagnosis of Stage III metastatic melanoma, Shannon was introduced to the possibility of joining a clinical trial testing the combination of relatlimab and nivolumab as a treatment before surgery. Her husband Rob was hesitant initially, worried about her being treated as a "guinea pig." However, after speaking with her doctors, Shannon embraced the trial, confident in its potential to help her fight this aggressive cancer.

Shannon's journey was not without its challenges. Her second infusion caused an allergic reaction, forcing adjustments to the treatment schedule. And as the COVID-19 pandemic began to unfold, Shannon faced further hurdles, including undergoing surgery alone and isolating from her family during recovery. Despite these obstacles, her treatment was a resounding success. Two rounds of therapy followed by surgery left Shannon with no evidence of disease. She went on to complete the full course of treatment, ringing a celebratory bell sent to her by a friend who had supported her every step of the way.

Shannon's experience underscores the profound potential of LAG-3-targeted therapies as a scientific breakthrough and a source of hope for people navigating some of life's toughest challenges. Despite hurdles, every step forward in understanding and targeting immune checkpoints like LAG-3 brings new opportunities for patients like Shannon to overcome the odds and live fuller lives.

Drug (Brand Name)	Target(s)	Initial U.S. Approval	Manufacturer	Notable Cancer Indication
nivolumab & relatlimab (Opdualag)	PD-1 & LAG-3	2022	Bristol-Myers Squibb	advanced melanoma

Figure 14. PD-1/LAG-3 Checkpoint Inhibitors. ACCESS HEALTH INTERNATIONAL

Checkpoint inhibitors have revolutionized cancer treatment, offering new hope to those with limited options. However, their true power lies in combination therapies, which unify the complementary strengths of approaches like chemotherapy, radiation, and checkpoint inhibitors. These pairings amplify the immune system's ability to target cancer, creating synergies that deliver more effective results. Yet, with this heightened power comes increased risk: higher toxicity and a greater chance of severe side effects. How do we strike the balance between efficacy and safety? In the next chapter, we'll revisit John Dabell's inspiring journey with head and neck cancer to explore the transformative promise—and the challenges—of combination therapies.

CHAPTER 6

Better Together —The Power of Combination Therapies

Back in Chapter II, we followed John Dabell's grueling battle with head and neck cancer—an ordeal that involved surgery, radiotherapy and chemotherapy. This trifecta of treatments kept the disease at bay for an astonishing eleven years, a length of remission some would call a cure. But the threat of relapse trails behind even long-term cancer survivors. A few rogue cells, too small to detect, can bide their time and return when least expected.

John was no exception. After years without symptoms, the labored breathing, white patches, and trouble swallowing were all too familiar. By the time doctors found the tumor—golf-ball-sized and menacing—it was clear the fight wasn't over.

While his first encounter with cancer saw surgery deliver the knockout blow, this time it wasn't enough. Chemotherapy helped temporarily, but the pandemic brought an abrupt end to his treatment, allowing the cancer to surge forward. Like sand slipping through his fingers, John felt his options slide out of reach.

John's story took a turn when he began a groundbreaking combination of high-dosage radiotherapy and nivolumab, a checkpoint inhibitor. Astonishingly, with this treatment duo, John's body began to fight back. The adverse effects he had braced for never materialized; instead, he grew stronger with each infusion.

Three years and 40 infusions later, John defied the odds, becoming a "super responder" to immunotherapy. His CT scans revealed no evidence of disease. Now, John visits the hospital once a month for his inhibitor infusion, a ritual he considers a “spa treatment” for the benefits it provides him. Once again, John could treasure the simple joys in his life—hiking in the tranquil hills of his hometown in Nottingham, writing on his online website, and spending precious time with his wife and daughter.

John’s second brush with cancer highlights the constant threat of recurrence. Tumors can return even after extensive bouts of treatment. Even worse, returning cancers often adapt, learning to resist the therapies used against them. Checkpoint inhibitors, for example, can lose effectiveness as tumors evolve to produce fewer of the immune checkpoints these therapies target.

This is where combination treatments come into play. By pairing therapies like surgery, chemotherapy, or radiation with immunotherapy—or even combining two immunotherapies—clinicians are crafting strategies that are greater than the sum of their parts. In this chapter, we’ll dive into some of the most promising combinations shaping the future of cancer care.

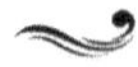

When it comes to cancer, a one-size-fits-all approach simply doesn’t cut it—especially when the disease has spread extensively. Rather than a single treatment, patients will often need a stack of therapies to build a multi-pronged approach, such as blending radiation with chemotherapy or using targeted drugs to pave the way for surgery. While a relatively new advance, checkpoint inhibitors have slotted into these traditional strategies with ease to create stronger and more effective treatments.

Surgery is a time-tested yet invasive, method for tackling cancers. This head-on approach often damages healthy tissues, and despite a surgeon's precision, stray cancer cells can sometimes evade the scalpel, lying in wait before returning with a vengeance. Here is where checkpoint inhibitors can shine. They can be given before surgery to whittle away at tumors and make them easier to remove. After surgery, these therapies can survey the body and eliminate any tumor cells left behind, thereby reducing the chances of recurrence. One melanoma study illustrates this post-operative benefit, as patients treated with inhibitor therapy after surgery saw their chances of staying recurrence-free improve by 40% compared to surgery alone.

Checkpoint inhibitors and chemotherapy make an unlikely yet powerful duo in the fight against cancer. Chemotherapy works by directly targeting rapidly dividing cells—damaging cancer cells but also affecting healthy tissue. While this can weaken the immune system overall, it also creates a window of opportunity for checkpoint inhibitors to step in.

As chemotherapy destroys cancer cells, it can release tumor antigens, essentially leaving a "breadcrumb trail" of identifiable proteins for the immune system. Immune cells can naturally detect and respond to these antigens, but their attack often falls short due to the cancer's ability to suppress immune activity. Checkpoint inhibitors can change this dynamic by lifting these hurdles and releasing T cells that the tumor's defensive checkpoints would otherwise silence.

Chemotherapy can also influence what immune cells enter the fray. These medicines disrupt pathways that suppress immune responses and eliminate certain immune cells that hinder T cell activity, such as regulatory T cells. Some chemotherapy drugs can even enhance T cell activation and promote the growth of specific T cells in patients with advanced cancers. Together, these treatments not only shrink tumors but also create a more hostile environment for cancer, with chemotherapy clearing the way and checkpoint inhibitors driving a sustained and targeted immune attack.

This synergy can help patients across multiple cancer types live longer, although the best results have been seen with lung cancers. According to meta-analysis data on non-small cell lung cancer, PD-1 or PD-L1 inhibitors with chemotherapy significantly reduce the risk of death compared to chemotherapy alone; most notably, patients on pembrolizumab combinations lived an average of 2.18 years longer than those on standard chemotherapy regimes over a five year period. For small cell lung cancer, a rare and aggressive form of lung cancer, three times more patients were alive at the three-year mark when treated with PD-L1 targeting durvalumab plus chemotherapy over chemotherapy alone. Other FDA-approved applications include small-cell lung cancer, triple-negative breast cancer, gastric and esophageal cancers, and cervical cancer, among others.

Survival Benefit of Checkpoint Inhibitor + Chemotherapy Treatments for nsNSCLC

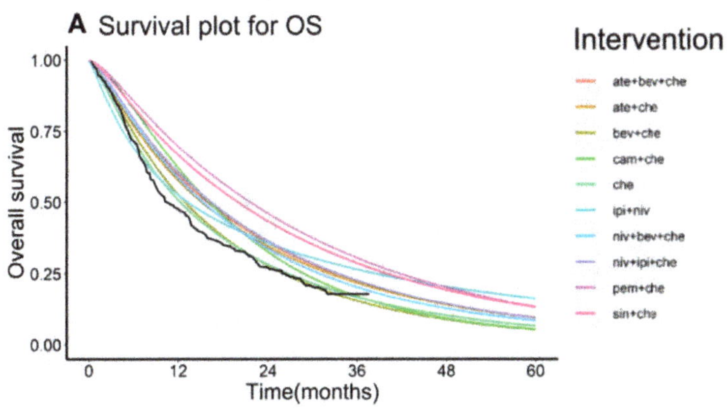

Figure 15. Overall Survival Plot of Several Checkpoint Inhibitor Plus Chemotherapy Combinations. The black line is the Kaplan-Meier (KM) curve for reference chemotherapy. [Abbreviations: ate+bev+che, atezolizumab+bevacizumab+chemotherapy; cam,camrelizumab; ipi, ipilimumab; niv, nivolumab; pem, pembrolizumab; sin, sintilimab]. SHAO, ZHAO, LIANG AND TANG (2022). FRONT. IMMUNOL.

Radiation therapy and checkpoint inhibitors are another compelling combination that harnesses the strengths of both approaches to deliver a one-two punch against cancer.

Radiation works by damaging the DNA of cancer cells, triggering their destruction. This process not only reduces tumor size but also releases tumor antigens—fragments of cancer cells that serve as beacons for the immune system. The flood of tumor antigens stimulates dendritic cells, which present these antigens to T cells, effectively training the immune system to recognize their enemy. Checkpoint inhibitors complement this process by preventing cancer cells from shutting off the T cells needed for the attack. This treatment duo primes the immune system and unravels its might in a single strike.

This strategy can yield positive results for patients with non-small cell lung cancer; one study found that patients who have previously undergone radiation and then checkpoint inhibitors experience longer overall survival than those treated with pembrolizumab alone. Another trial on urothelial cancer suggests that a history of radiotherapy may be an essential factor in achieving more prolonged survival on pembrolizumab. However, there is room to assess the best dose of radiotherapy needed for each patient and determine a standard for when checkpoint inhibitors should be taken after radiotherapy.

Targeted drugs are another class of cancer treatment that complements checkpoint inhibitors. While these medicines disrupt critical cancer pathways by honing in on specific molecules that fuel tumor growth and survival, checkpoint inhibitors amplify the immune system's ability to detect and destroy cancer cells.

One of the most compelling examples of this synergy is angiogenesis inhibitors, which block the growth of new blood vessels that tumors need to survive. Pairing these drugs with checkpoint inhibitors has shown impressive outcomes in several cancers. For instance, combining the angiogenesis inhibitor axitinib with the PD-1 inhibitor pembrolizumab in advanced renal cell carcinoma led to a median progression-free survival of 15.1 months compared to 11.1 months with pembrolizumab alone. This combination also improved overall response rates, demonstrating how these therapies can complement one another.

Other targeted therapies, such as PARP inhibitors and MAPK/ERK pathway inhibitors, are also being investigated in combination with checkpoint inhibitors. PARP inhibitors, often used in BRCA-mutated cancers, can increase DNA damage in cancer cells, making them more visible to the immune system and enhancing the effects of checkpoint inhibitors. Meanwhile, targeting the MAPK/ERK pathway—commonly activated in melanoma and other cancers—can help dismantle tumor defenses, paving the way for an improved immune attack.

In the ever-evolving chess match against cancer, we attempt to predict our opponent's moves—usually to limited success. Even though we try our best to outmaneuver cancer with combination treatments, they are far from a universal solution.

Chemotherapy often depletes the immune system, paradoxically reducing the immune force that checkpoint inhibitors aim to bolster. Radiation, though precise, can trigger inflammatory responses that actually can suppress immune reactivity. Surgery can create localized trauma that temporarily dampens immune surveillance. And even targeted drugs, designed to attack specific molecular pathways, can create resistance mechanisms that render checkpoint therapies less effective.

Moreover, this stronger offensive comes with a heavier toll on the body. For instance, checkpoint inhibitors with chemotherapy frequently lead to increased fatigue, nausea, and a heightened risk of infection. Similarly, radiation combined with checkpoint therapy can exacerbate inflammation, leading to severe pneumonitis in some cases. This poses challenges for patients and clinicians alike.

Looking forward, the key might lie in novel strategies: testing combinations beyond two therapies, such as inhibitor therapy after chemoradiation, experimenting with sequencing and personalizing regimens to individual cancer profiles. Future research could unlock a blueprint for treatments that perfectly balance potency and safety.

Stand-alone checkpoint inhibitors can prolong survival for some patients with hard-to-treat cancers—no small feat by any means. Yet, these therapies remain far from universal in their effectiveness. Most patients either do not respond from the start or experience relapse as their cancers evolve resistance. This underscores an urgent need to improve both the initial effectiveness of checkpoint inhibitors and the durability of their results.

To turn the tide, researchers have found that combining checkpoint inhibitors can unlock new possibilities. Confronting two distinct but complementary immune pathways can enhance T cell activation compared to tackling a single pathway alone. This approach boosts antitumor responses and offers a critical advantage: it may help patients overcome resistance to single-agent therapies, broadening the reach of immunotherapy's benefits.

A familiar example is **Opdulag**, a checkpoint inhibitor that is pre-mixed with PD-1 and LAG-3 targeting antibodies. Melanoma patients on this combined infusion experience improved survival over those on PD-1 targeting nivolumab alone. In a follow-up study, Opdulag continues to provide a survival benefit even three years after treatment, with almost 49% of patients alive at the study's end-mark versus around 39% of patients on PD-1 monotherapy.

CTLA-4 and PD-1 inhibitor combinations, such as ipilimumab and nivolumab from Bristol-Meyer Squibb or tremelimumab and durvalumab from AstraZeneca, have become a focal point in cancer immunotherapy research. These pairings take advantage of complementary mechanisms to maximize immune activation. For ipilimumab and nivolumab, treatment usually begins with CTLA-4 blockade to bolster T cell activation in lymph nodes, followed by PD-1 inhibition to sustain and refine immune responses beyond the immune organs. In contrast, tremelimumab and durvalumab are often administered as an initial combined dose to jumpstart immune activation before continuing with the PD-1 inhibitor.

This combined attack helps the immune system produce more of the signal molecules T cells need to communicate effectively and decreases the ratio of regulatory T cells (Tregs) to our active fighting T cells, such as killer T cells. This is important because having fewer immunosuppressive Tregs means that the immune system can be more active against cancer. Visualize regulatory T cells as coaches who tell a team of immune cell players to sit on the bench. If fewer players sit out, more can help win the game against cancer. Altogether, these dual CTLA-4/PD-1 strategies amplify T cell numbers and activity, overwhelming tumors with an immune attack on multiple fronts.

Combining CTLA-4 and PD-1 inhibitors produces significant survival advantages over using either therapy alone, particularly for cancers like melanoma and non-small cell lung cancer (NSCLC). In advanced melanoma, a groundbreaking study revealed that nearly half of all patients treated with nivolumab and ipilimumab were alive 6.5 years after starting therapy. When compared to just

34% of patients who received nivolumab alone and 22% on ipilimumab monotherapy.

Combination therapy outperforms chemotherapy, a standard first-line treatment for people with non-small cell lung cancer. As shown in the figure below, 42% of patients on the dual regimen were still alive five years after treatment compared to only 28% on chemotherapy. What makes this approach even more promising is its versatility. Unlike PD-1 inhibitors alone, this dual-inhibitor therapy delivers results regardless of PD-L1 expression, ensuring more patients have access to its life-extending potential.

CTLA-4/PD-1 Blockade V.S. Chemotherapy for NSCLC

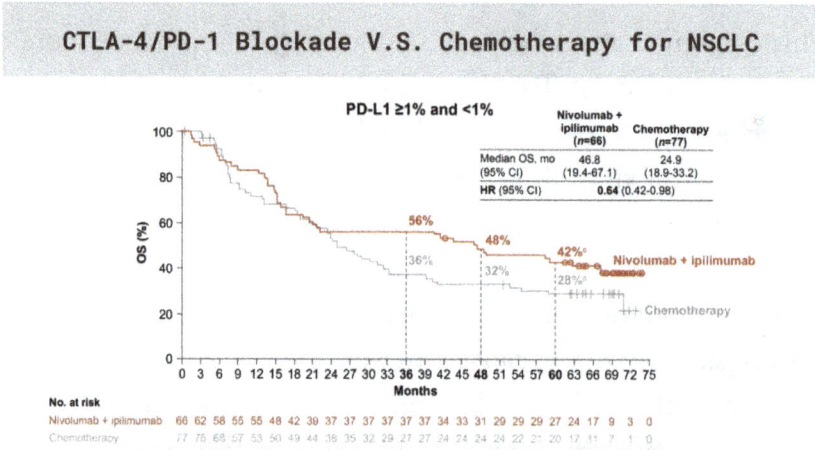

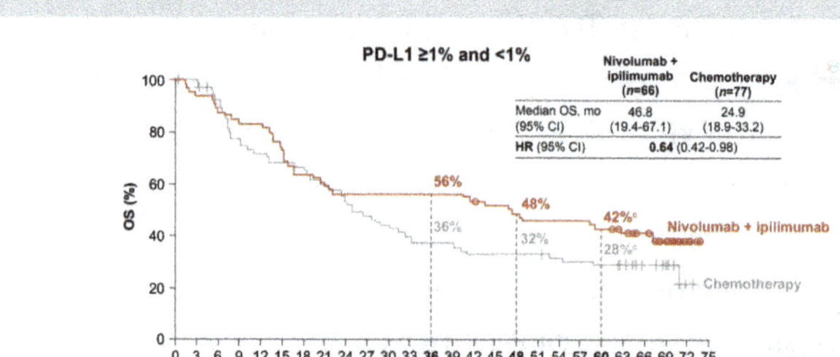

Figure 16. Overall Survival in Japanese Patients with Metastatic Non-Small Cell Lung Cancer (NSCLC). Graph combines results for patients with low (PD-L1<1%) vs high (PD-L1≥ 1%) PD-L1 tumor expression. NISHIO, M., OHE, Y., IKEDA, S. ET AL. (2023). INT J CLIN ONCOL.

Despite these encouraging results, the CTLA-4/PD-1 pairing is not universally beneficial. In some cases, such as with advanced melanoma that has spread to the mucus membranes of the body, the combination offers similar efficacy to PD-1 monotherapy but with higher rates of unwanted adverse immune effects. Furthermore, real-world data suggests that this combination may be most beneficial for patients with multi-organ metastasis, while PD-1 monotherapy is likely best for those whose cancer is present in only one or two organs.

The pairing of PD-1 and PD-L1 inhibitors sits at the crossroads of promise and debate. Each treatment represents a key to the same lock; if both target the same immune pathway, is it worth using them together? Some scientists say that blocking PD-1, PD-L1, and PD-L2 interactions at once could release a torrent of immune activity. Others counter that PD-1 inhibitors alone already accomplish this by targeting multiple ligands.

An alternative option is to use a staggered approach: starting with a PD-L1 inhibitor and following-up with PD-1 therapy. Some tumors adapt to PD-L1 treatment by expressing more PD-L2 checkpoints on their surface, allowing them to hide from the immune system. A PD-1 inhibitor could counter this evasive maneuver. Yet, clinical data remains inconclusive. Patients with advanced renal cell carcinoma showed limited benefits from sequential PD-1/PD-L1 therapy compared to PD-1 monotherapy.

Even when dual therapies work, they come with a price. As more T cells spring into action, the risk of dangerous inflammation grows. This is why severe immune-related adverse effects occur at far higher rates with combined inhibitor therapies than with single inhibitors. For example, a comparative study on advanced melanoma found that more than twice as many patients on combined CTLA-4/PD-1 therapy experienced severe immune reactions than those on PD-1 monotherapy (about 34% to 12%).

Balancing efficacy and safety is paramount; for some patients, sticking to monotherapy might be the wiser route.

Importantly, dual inhibitor therapy can extend survival and deliver remarkable outcomes, it doesn't eliminate the risk of recurrence. When this happens, switching strategies may open new doors. Experimenting with a different checkpoint combination as a second-line treatment, such as PD-1/LAG-3 after CTLA-4/PD-1, could yield interesting results but more research is needed.

Dual-inhibitor strategies push the frontiers of immunotherapy, building on the successes of single-agent therapies to deliver impressive results. At the same time, the heightened antitumor response of these pairings comes with its own challenges, such as navigating more severe immune-related adverse events and ongoing uncertainties. This balance between potency and safety will remain a focal point as applications for these treatments grow and new combinations come to the fore.

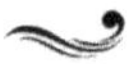

Beyond conventional cancer therapies, researchers continue to test the waters with fresh therapy combinations, including integrating inhibitors with new experimental checkpoints, cancer-targeting viruses, and tumor vaccines. With this momentum, two immunotherapy giants could one day join forces: checkpoint inhibitors and another revolutionary immunotherapy known as CAR T therapy.

Chimeric Antigen T Cell Therapy is a cancer advance that cleverly fuses the targeting power of antibodies with the cancer-killing machinery of a T cell. The process uses gene editing to alter a patient's extracted T cells, equipping them with synthetic receptors before returning them to the body. The new receptors give the T cells a superior ability to hone in and eliminate tumor cells—a strategy that can successfully treat hard-to-treat blood cancers like multiple myeloma but is also susceptible to exhaustion. This is where checkpoint inhibitors can step in to synergize.

Checkpoint inhibitors offer a powerful boost to CAR T therapies breathing life back into exhausted T cells that lost their fight against tumors. in studies on diffuse large B-cell lymphoma, adding PD-1 targeting pembrolizumab after CAR T therapy re-expanded CAR T cell populations in eight out of 11 patients with progressive disease, effectively giving the immune system a second wind. Moreover, simultaneous checkpoint blockade shields CAR T cells from cancer's ploys, such as overexpressing PD-L1 and PD-L2 to shut down CAR T cell activity; a trial showed a 72% response rate in mesothelioma patients treated with CAR T cells and anti-PD-1 agents, highlighting the untapped possibilities of this synergy.

Checkpoint inhibitors also help CAR T cells live longer, creating sustained responses. The timing must be carefully orchestrated, as patients who receive the inhibitor within weeks of their CAR T infusion typically yield better results.

Perhaps most exciting is the opportunity to bring CAR T therapies to a new territory: treating solid tumors. Historically, these interventions have been unable to the tumor microenvironment (TME), which acts as a fortress shielding cancer from immune attack. Checkpoint inhibitors can empower the immune system to pierce these defenses, creating a foothold for CAR T cells to operate more effectively. Early clinical trials for solid tumors like glioblastoma demonstrate the approach is feasible and safe, but more data is needed to establish safety and efficacy.

The power of checkpoint inhibitor combinations lies in their ability to transform the fight against cancer, pushing the scales back in the patient's favor. However, this power comes with a price. For many, the trade-off for improved outcomes is the risk of severe toxicities. The key to unlocking their full personalization—much like crafting a tailored suit for each patient, we must match the right strategy to the right individual. Continued research will finetune this delicate balancing act, unlocking new combined interventions that extend survival and preserve the quality of life.

CHAPTER 7

Hit or Miss — The Effects of Checkpoint Inhibitors

The essence of our current struggle with checkpoint inhibitor therapy is that they are a revolution in some cancers, a disappointment in others. But why? What distinguishes the winners from the defeated in this molecular battle?

Let's start with a surprising underdog: Merkel cell carcinoma. Never heard of it? You're not alone. This rare skin cancer, while not as well-known as its cousins melanoma or basal cell carcinoma, is not to be underestimated.

Merkel cell carcinoma (MCC) occurs when these touch-sensing cells mutate and start to multiply uncontrollably. The cells form a hard, raised, reddish-purplish bump that seems to appear out of nowhere and grows at an alarming rate.

What makes this cancer particularly sneaky is its origin story. In about 80% of cases, a virus called Merkel cell polyomavirus (MCPyV) is the culprit. This virus, harmless to most, can sometimes hijack the genetic machinery of Merkel cells, turning them into cancerous troublemakers. The remaining 20% of cases are linked to damage from ultraviolet radiation, much like a sunburn gone terribly wrong.

Once these rogue cells take hold, they don't play nice. This cancer is known to spreading quickly and aggressively to nearby lymph nodes. Then, in their hostile takeover, the tumor cells use the lymph vessels as highways to invade new territories.

This rare skin cancer was once a death sentence, with most patients surviving less than a year after diagnosis. Survival rates skyrocketed as checkpoint inhibitors burst into the scene. Up to 70% of patients now respond to treatment, with many enjoying long-term remission.

But for every Merkel cell carcinoma, there's a pancreatic cancer—stubbornly resistant to checkpoint inhibition. Despite billions invested in research, pancreatic cancer remains one of the deadliest malignancies, with checkpoint inhibitors showing little effect in most patients.

The stark differences in treatment outcomes can be attributed to the intricate details of tumor biology. To illustrate, we can imagine two fortresses. One is made of glass, with transparent and fragile defenses. The other is a stone behemoth with thick and impenetrable walls. Our checkpoint inhibitor army might easily breach the glass fortress, but it would barely scratch the stone one.

Merkel cell carcinoma is our glass fortress. It's often caused by a virus, making it look foreign to our immune system. It also tends to have a high mutation load, providing plenty of "flags" for our immune cells to recognize.

Pancreatic cancer, on the other hand, is our stone fortress. It creates a dense, fibrous shield around itself and employs various tricks to keep immune cells at bay. This fortress lies tucked away behind your stomach that normally helps with digestion and blood sugar control.

But when cancer takes hold, it transforms this helpful organ into a stronghold of disease.

At the heart of this fortress are the cancer cells themselves, often kickstarted by a mutation in a gene called KRAS13. Think of KRAS as the castle's power source—when it goes haywire, it keeps the lights on 24/7, driving relentless growth and division. As the cancer progresses, it accumulates more genetic changes, like adding towers and battlements to its defenses.

What makes pancreatic cancer truly formidable is its ability to recruit allies. It doesn't just build walls; it creates an entire hostile landscape around itself. The cancer cells summon pancreatic stellate cells, normally tasked with tissue repair, and push them into overdrive. These corrupted helpers produce a thick, protein-rich goo that envelops the tumor like a moat, creating an almost impenetrable barrier against drugs and immune cells.

But the cancer's ingenuity doesn't stop there. It disrupts the formation of blood vessels, resulting in a chaotic vascular system that acts like a faulty drawbridge. This haphazard network limits the flow of oxygen, nutrients, and crucially, cancer-fighting agents to the tumor site. As if these physical defenses weren't enough, pancreatic cancer is also a master of disguise. It often presents fewer mutations than other cancers, giving the immune system fewer "flags" to recognize - it's as if the entire castle is painted to blend seamlessly into the surrounding landscape.

The cancer doesn't just defend; it actively recruits allies. It sends out chemical signals that lure immune cells, only to reprogram them upon arrival. These turncoat cells, instead of attacking, end up protecting the tumor and even aiding its growth. It's a brilliant strategy of turning potential enemies into loyal guards. And as a final, insidious tactic, pancreatic cancer is notorious for sending out scouts early. Even small tumors can dispatch cellular emissaries throughout the body, establishing distant outposts in other organs, often before the primary tumor is even detected. This multi-pronged approach transforms the pancreas from a vital organ into a veritable stronghold of disease, explaining why this particular cancer has proven so resistant to our current arsenal of treatments.

This multi-layered defense system explains why pancreatic cancer is so resistant to our current treatments. Chemotherapy struggles to breach the walls, targeted therapies find their targets hidden or changed, and immunotherapies face an environment actively working against them. It's as if we're trying to storm a fortress with medieval weapons against modern defenses.

But in the complex world of cancer, even the most formidable fortresses can have hidden weaknesses. Sometimes, what appears to be an impenetrable stone wall might conceal a secret passage. This brings us to an intriguing contrast: colorectal cancer.

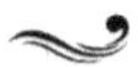

At first glance, colorectal cancer seems to share pancreatic cancer's stone fortress qualities, often proving resistant to checkpoint inhibition. But a closer inspection reveals a chink in its armor. About 5% of colorectal cancers have a specific genetic signature called microsatellite instability-high (MSI-H). For patients with this subtype, it's as if we've discovered a hidden key to the castle gates.

Checkpoint inhibitors, largely ineffective against other colorectal cancers, can be remarkably potent for these MSI-H tumors.

The reason for this effectiveness as explained by Dana-Farber's Benjamin L. Schlechter, MD, "Because MSI-H colorectal cancers have a large number of genetic mutations, it's relatively easy for the immune system to find abnormalities on tumor cells that it can latch onto and attack. The more normal-appearing nature of MSS cancers, however, makes them less visible to the immune system. As a result, MSS tumors don't respond as well to immunotherapy."

This striking difference illustrates a crucial lesson in modern oncology: the devil—and sometimes the angel—is in the details. Understanding the distinct genetic and molecular characteristics of each tumor can unveil unexpected vulnerabilities, turning seemingly impregnable fortresses into conquerable targets.

This complexity raises a critical question: How can we determine which patients benefit from checkpoint inhibitors? This question keeps oncologists up at night and motivates researchers to delve even deeper into the genetic and molecular foundations of cancer.

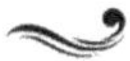

Biomarkers offer one potential answer. These biological signposts might indicate whether a tumor will respond to checkpoint inhibition. PD-L1 expression is one such marker, but it's far from perfect.

PD-L1, or Programmed Death-Ligand 1, is like an invisibility cloak that some cancer cells wear. When a T cell encounters a cell displaying PD-L1, it receives a "stand down" signal. This interaction tricks the T cell into ignoring the cancer cell, allowing the tumor to grow unchecked.

Checkpoint inhibitors are drugs designed to block this interaction, essentially stripping away the cancer's invisibility cloak and allowing T cells to recognize and attack the tumor; therefore PD-L1 expression on tumor cells can be measured and used as a biomarker to predict how well a patient might respond to these drugs. High PD-L1 expression often suggests a better chance of response to checkpoint inhibitors. The logic is straightforward: if a tumor is relying heavily on PD-L1 to evade the immune system, then blocking this pathway should be particularly effective.

However, the relationship between PD-L1 expression and treatment response isn't always clear-cut. Some tumors with high PD-L1 expression don't respond to treatment. Conversely, some tumors with low or no detectable PD-L1 still benefit from checkpoint inhibitors.

The complexity of PD-L1 as a biomarker is evident across various cancer types. In melanoma, renal cell carcinoma, non-small cell lung cancer, and bladder cancer—cancers where checkpoint inhibitors have shown remarkable success—PD-L1 expression can range from as low as 14% to as high as 100% of tumor samples. This wide variability highlights the challenges in using PD-L1 as a definitive predictor of treatment response.

Consider non-small cell lung cancer, where PD-L1 testing has become a standard part of treatment decision-making. Patients with high PD-L1 expression, 50% or more of tumor cells, are usually given checkpoint inhibitors rather than traditional chemotherapy or combination therapies. However, even patients with lower or no

PD-L1 expression can sometimes benefit, making treatment decisions complex.

Also, it is critical to note that cancer's interaction with the immune system involves many factors beyond just PD-L1. Other elements of the tumor microenvironment, genetic factors, and even the patient's overall health can influence treatment response.

The search for better biomarkers continues, driven by the need to more accurately predict who will benefit from these powerful but potentially toxic treatments. Tumor mutational burden (TMB) is one promising avenue. TMB measures the number of mutations in a tumor's DNA. Higher TMB often correlates with better responses to immunotherapy, possibly because more mutations create more "foreign-looking" proteins that the immune system can recognize.

The search for better biomarkers continues, driven by the need to more accurately predict who will benefit from these powerful but potentially toxic treatments. The makeup of specific immune cells in the tumor microenvironment (TME) is an area of intense study, as these cells play a critical role in determining how well a patient's cancer will respond to treatments like checkpoint inhibitors. The TME consists not only of cancer cells but also of various immune cells, blood vessels, and supporting structures that interact with each other in complex ways.

One key player is the T cell, a type of white blood cell that is essential for the immune response. There are different types of T cells, and their presence and activity within the tumor can significantly influence treatment outcomes. For example, cytotoxic T cells, also known as CD8+ T cells, are responsible for directly attacking and killing cancer cells. The higher the density of these cytotoxic T cells within a tumor, the more likely it is that the tumor will respond to immunotherapy. Studies have shown that tumors with a robust infiltration of CD8+ T cells often correlate with better patient prognosis and improved responses to checkpoint inhibitors.

In addition to cytotoxic T cells, helper T cells (CD4+ T cells) also play a crucial role in orchestrating the immune response. They help activate other immune cells, including B cells and additional T cells, enhancing the overall immune attack against tumors. Certain subtypes of helper T cells, such as Th1 cells, are particularly effective at promoting anti-tumor immunity by producing cytokines that stimulate CD8+ T cell activity.

However, not all immune cells within the TME are beneficial. Regulatory T cells, for example, can suppress the immune response and create an environment that allows tumors to thrive. An abundance of Tregs can hinder the effectiveness of checkpoint inhibitors by dampening the activity of cytotoxic T cells. Therefore, understanding the balance between pro-tumor and anti-tumor immune populations is vital for predicting treatment responses.

Research has shown that specific patterns of immune cell infiltration can serve as biomarkers for treatment response. For instance, tumors characterized by high levels of CD8+ T cell infiltration and low levels of Tregs tend to have better responses to checkpoint inhibitors. Conversely, tumors with a predominance of immunosuppressive cell types may be less responsive to these therapies.

Intriguingly, the makeup of a patient's gut microbiome—the vast collection of bacteria and other microorganisms residing in our digestive tract—is emerging as a fascinating area of research in the quest to predict responses to immunotherapy. This collection of microbes plays a crucial role in our overall health, influencing everything from digestion to immune function. Recent studies suggest that the diversity and composition of these gut bacteria might significantly impact how well patients respond to treatments like checkpoint inhibitors, which are designed to unleash the immune system against cancer.

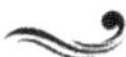

The intestinal microbiome is teeming with diverse inhabitants—some friendly and helpful, others harmful or indifferent. A portion of this microbial community interacts closely with your immune system, helping it recognize and respond to threats such as cancer cells. When integrating immunotherapies such as checkpoint inhibitors, the composition of this microbial city can influence how effectively the immune system mounts an attack against tumors.

Research has shown that patients with a more diverse gut microbiome—meaning a wider variety of bacterial species—tend to have better outcomes when treated with immunotherapy. This diversity is thought to enhance the immune response by providing a richer array of signals that can activate immune cells. For instance, certain beneficial bacteria can produce metabolites that stimulate the immune system or help train T cells to recognize and attack cancer cells more effectively.

Not all bacteria are created equal in this context. Some studies have identified specific bacterial species that appear to correlate with positive responses to checkpoint inhibitors. For example, *Akkermansia muciniphila* and *Bifidobacterium longum* have been associated with improved treatment outcomes. These "good" bacteria seem to help prime the immune system, making it more effective at targeting tumors.

Conversely, some bacterial species may hinder treatment effectiveness. Certain "bad" bacteria can interfere with immune cell function or promote inflammation in ways that are detrimental to the body's ability to fight cancer. This complex interplay between different types of bacteria underscores the need for a deeper understanding of how our gut microbiome influences cancer treatment.

How exactly does the gut microbiome affect immunotherapy responses? One theory suggests that beneficial bacteria can enhance the production of short-chain fatty acids (SCFAs), which are metabolites produced during the fermentation of dietary fibers. SCFAs play a vital role in regulating immune responses and may help boost the activity of T cells involved in attacking tumors.

Moreover, researchers are exploring how changes in the gut microbiome before and during treatment can provide insights into patient outcomes. By analyzing stool samples from patients undergoing immunotherapy, scientists can identify patterns in microbial composition that correlate with treatment success or failure.

As research continues to unfold, there is growing interest in potentially manipulating the gut microbiome as a strategy for enhancing immunotherapy effectiveness. Approaches such as probiotics or dietary interventions aimed at increasing beneficial bacteria could become part of personalized treatment plans for cancer patients. The idea is not just about identifying which bacteria are present but also about fostering an environment within the gut that supports a robust immune response.

By delving deeper into cancer biology, it's become clear that no single biomarker will likely be sufficient to predict treatment response across all patients and cancer types. The future of cancer therapy may lie in combining multiple biomarkers to create a more comprehensive picture of each patient's unique tumor landscape.

This personalized approach, often referred to as precision oncology, aims to match the right treatment to the right patient at the right time. While challenges remain, the ongoing research into biomarkers offers hope for more effective, tailored cancer treatments in the future.

Importantly, patients whose cancers do not respond to current checkpoint inhibitors are not necessarily left behind in this immunotherapy revolution. Instead, they represent a critical area of focus for researchers and clinicians who are committed to expanding the benefits of immunotherapy to a broader range of patients.

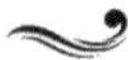

Researchers are investigating different methods to transform "cold" tumors, which do not attract immune cells, into "hot" tumors that may be responsive to checkpoint inhibition. These methods include combining checkpoint inhibitors with other treatments and creating entirely new categories of immunotherapy drugs.

Jeffrey Hubbell, the Eugene Bell Professor in Tissue Engineering at University of Chicago offers this perspective: "Once we have a way to make a cold tumor hot, the possibilities for cancer treatment are endless."

To grasp the significance of transforming cold tumors into hot ones, it's essential to understand what these terms mean in the context of cancer. Cold tumors are characterized by a lack of immune cell infiltration; they remain largely unrecognized by the immune system. This absence of immune activity allows these tumors to grow and spread without being challenged. In contrast, hot tumors are teeming with immune cells actively engaging with the tumor, making them more susceptible to immunotherapy.

The transformation of cold tumors into hot tumors involves several scientific strategies designed to stimulate an immune response. A primary goal is to create an inflammatory environment within the tumor, which can be achieved through various means. One effective approach is the use of cytokines—proteins that mediate and regulate immunity and inflammation. For instance, interleukin-12 (IL-12) is a powerful cytokine known for its ability to recruit immune cells to the tumor site. By delivering IL-12 directly to cold tumors, researchers can provoke an inflammatory response that attracts T cells and other immune components.

In addition to cytokines, the tumor microenvironment plays a crucial role in determining whether a tumor is classified as cold or hot. Another innovative strategy involves the use of oncolytic viruses—viruses that selectively infect and kill cancer cells while simultaneously stimulating an immune response. These viruses can help convert cold tumors into hot ones by inducing cell death and releasing tumor antigens that draw immune cells to the area.

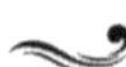

Moreover, advanced drug delivery systems utilizing nanoparticles are being developed to target therapies directly to tumors. These nanoparticles can encapsulate drugs or cytokines and release them specifically at the tumor site, minimizing systemic side effects while maximizing local immune activation. Together, these approaches represent a multifaceted strategy to enhance the immune response against previously unresponsive tumors, paving the way for more effective cancer treatments.

Transforming cold tumors into hot ones holds immense promise for expanding the effectiveness of immunotherapy across a broader range of cancers. By making previously unresponsive tumors visible to the immune system, researchers aim to unlock new treatment options for patients who currently have limited choices.

The implications of this research are profound. If successful, these strategies could lead to breakthroughs in treating aggressive cancers that have historically been resistant to conventional therapies. For patients with cold tumors—such as certain types of breast cancer or pancreatic cancer—this transformation could mean access to life-saving treatments that harness their own immune systems in ways never before possible.

Checkpoint inhibitors have rewritten the rules of engagement for some cancers, offering hope where once there was none. But they've also revealed the staggering complexity of our enemy, showing us just how much we still have to learn.

One thing is sure: the era of immunotherapy is just beginning. And with it comes the promise of a future where cancer is not an implacable foe but a beatable one. A future where more patients can look forward to not just survival but life after cancer. The battle continues. But we can see a path to victory for the first time in decades. And that, perhaps, is the most significant victory of all.

PART III

Innovation, the Promising Road Ahead

CHAPTER 8

Tomorrow's Targets — Charting New Frontiers in Immunotherapy

It's now time to leave behind familiar terrain. Beyond the well-trodden path of CTLA-4, PD-1/PD-L1 and LAG-3 inhibitors stretches a vast, unexplored wilderness brimming with untapped potential. This realm is filled with cutting-edge ways to identifying cancers, novel checkpoints, innovative combinations, and groundbreaking approaches that promise to redefine the limits of cancer immunotherapy. This is a frontier where hope meets ingenuity, where the quest to cure cancer takes on an exhilarating new dimension.

In the relentless pursuit of early cancer detection, scientists are turning to blood tests to transform how we diagnose and treat this formidable disease. At the forefront of this scientific revolution are liquid biopsies and multi-cancer detection (MCD) tests, ingenious tools that can uncover the whispers of cancer long before symptoms appear. With this technology, a simple blood draw could reveal the presence of dozens of different cancers, all from a single sample.

Liquid biopsies and MCD tests act as molecular detectives, searching for telltale signs of cancer amidst the complex symphony of our blood. Just as fishing nets are cast wide, these tests catch variety of cancer signals that might otherwise slip through the cracks of conventional screening methods.

At the heart of these innovative approaches lies a sophisticated analysis of various biological signals that cancer leaves behind. As tumors grow and evolve, they shed molecular breadcrumbs into the bloodstream—circulating tumor cells (CTCs), circulating tumor DNA (ctDNA), fragments of RNA, and proteins that carry the unique signatures of cancer. Liquid biopsies and MCD tests are designed to detect and decipher these cryptic messages.

One of the key targets for these tests are changes in DNA and RNA sequences. Cancer is, at its core, a disease of altered genes, and these genetic changes can be detected in the fragments of DNA and RNA that circulate in our blood. By identifying specific mutations or alterations associated with various cancer types, these tests can raise red flags for further investigation.

Another powerful indicator that these tests look for are patterns of **DNA methylation**. Methylation is like a chemical switch that can turn genes on or off, and cancer cells often display abnormal methylation patterns. By mapping these epigenetic changes, liquid biopsies and MCD tests can spot the fingerprints of cancer even when the DNA sequence itself remains unchanged. The tests also examine DNA fragmentation patterns, as the way DNA breaks apart in cancer cells can differ from healthy cells. This fragmentation analysis adds another layer of detection, helping to distinguish between benign and malignant conditions.

With just 5 milliliters of blood—about a teaspoon—doctors can potentially detect a range of cancers, monitor treatment effectiveness, and even predict disease progression. The implications are staggering: earlier detection, personalized treatment plans, and real-time monitoring of cancer's molecular evolution.

As these technologies continue to evolve and improve, they paint a picture of a future where cancer detection becomes more precise, less invasive, and more widely accessible. The development of liquid biopsies and MCD tests represents a significant leap forward in our ability to outsmart cancer, offering new hope in the ongoing battle against this complex and formidable foe.

The innovations don't stop there. Scientists are also exploring the realm of synthetic biopsies, a technique that sounds like science fiction but holds immense potential. This approach aims to coax cancer cells out of hiding, forcing them to reveal themselves even in the disease's earliest stages. By manipulating the body's own processes, researchers hope to create a biological spotlight that illuminates cancerous cells, making them impossible to miss.

Artificial intelligence (AI) is also making its mark in cancer screening, bringing the power of machine learning to bear against this complex disease. AI algorithms are being trained to analyze mammograms with superhuman precision, potentially catching breast cancers that human eyes might miss. In regions lacking expert radiologists, AI could scan countless X-rays to flag potential concerns for further review.

Perhaps most remarkably, MIT's 'Sybil' AI model is pushing the boundaries of predictive medicine. By analyzing low-dose CT scans, Sybil can peer into the future, assessing an individual's risk of developing lung cancer up to six years in advance. This crystal ball of cancer detection could revolutionize how we approach prevention and early intervention, potentially saving countless lives.

The Cancer Screening Research Network (CSRN) is launching clinical trials to rigorously evaluate these emerging screening methods. Of particular interest are **multi-cancer detection tests**, which hold the promise of screening for multiple cancer types with a single blood draw. These trials will help separate hype from reality, ensuring that only the most effective and reliable screening tools make their way into clinical practice.

The future of cancer screening shines with promise and potential. From liquid biopsies that turn blood into a diagnostic powerhouse to AI models that predict cancer risk years in advance, these approaches bring us closer to a world where cancer can be caught early, treated effectively, and perhaps one day, prevented entirely.

As we've journeyed through this book, we've uncovered the intricate and deceptive nature of cancer, a true master of disguise. Like a skilled magician, it employs a myriad of strategies to elude our immune system, weaving a complex web that allows tumors to thrive and expand while remaining largely undetected by the body's vigilant defenses.

In response to this cunning adversary, researchers are shifting their focus from direct attacks on cancer cells to a more nuanced approach: releasing all the "brakes" on our immune system. This innovative strategy lies at the heart of multi-checkpoint targeting, which seeks to enhance the immune response against tumors by simultaneously inhibiting various checkpoint pathways. By unshackling the immune system from its constraints, we aim to empower it to recognize and destroy cancer cells more effectively, turning the tide in this relentless battle.

Compellingly, multi-checkpoint targeting dismantles the protective shield that cancers create by simultaneously blocking multiple checkpoints. We are beginning to understand that different immune checkpoints play distinct roles in immune suppression. By effectively targeting these pathways together, we have the potential to overcome resistance mechanisms and promote longer-lasting responses in cancer treatment.

This approach can be likened to removing several locks from a door that has been bolted shut. By disabling multiple inhibitory pathways at once, researchers aim to unleash a more robust immune response—one that can recognize and destroy cancer cells that have previously evaded detection. In doing so, multi-checkpoint targeting not only enhances the effectiveness of immunotherapy but also opens new avenues for combating resilient tumors.

One of the remarkable aspects of multi-checkpoint targeting is its ability to produce synergistic effects. This means that when multiple immune checkpoints are targeted simultaneously, the combined impact can be significantly greater than the sum of their individual effects. For instance, clinical trials have shown promising results when combining PD-1 inhibitors with CTLA-4 inhibitors in various cancers. This combination enhances T cell activation and proliferation, effectively boosting the immune response against tumors. By simultaneously blocking these checkpoints, researchers can reduce the immunosuppressive signals within the tumor microenvironment, allowing T cells to function more effectively.

Another critical advantage of multi-checkpoint targeting is its potential to overcome resistance. Many patients initially respond well to checkpoint inhibitors. Yet over time, their tumors can adapt and find ways to evade immune detection. For example, tumors can express more checkpoint proteins to continue shutting down the immune system, all while downregulating immune checkpoints that the patient's therapy actually targets. This phenomenon is known as acquired resistance.

Multi-checkpoint targeting aims to address this challenge by preventing tumors from developing new strategies to escape immune surveillance. By attacking multiple pathways involved in immune suppression, this approach seeks to keep the immune system engaged and capable of recognizing and attacking cancer cells more effectively.

Engaging multiple pathways involved in immune regulation through multi-checkpoint targeting may also lead to more durable responses in patients. A durable response means that not only can tumors be effectively attacked, but there is also a reduced chance of recurrence. By maintaining a vigilant immune system that continues to recognize and respond to any remaining cancer cells, patients may experience longer-lasting remissions. This aspect is particularly important in cancer treatment, as it offers hope for improved long-term outcomes and better quality of life for patients who have undergone therapy.

The clinical implications of multi-checkpoint targeting are profound. Researchers are actively investigating various combinations of checkpoint inhibitors in clinical trials, seeking to identify optimal pairings that maximize therapeutic efficacy while minimizing side effects. Early results have shown promise in treating cancers such as melanoma, lung cancer, and bladder cancer.

Multi-checkpoint targeting represents a significant advance in cancer immunotherapy. It offers hope for patients whose cancers have resisted traditional treatments, paving the way for more effective and personalized therapies.

Experimental antibodies in cancer treatment are microscopic guided missiles, exquisitely designed to seek and destroy cancer cells while leaving healthy cells unscathed. These molecular marvels are painstakingly crafted in laboratories, often inspired by the immune systems of patients who have successfully battled cancer. In a process that sounds like science fiction, researchers isolate millions of immune cells from these survivors, screening them for the perfect cancer-fighting antibodies. Through a series of rigorous tests, they whittle down the candidates until they find the most potent cancer-killers.

An exciting approach in this arena is the development of **bispecific antibodies**. These molecular marvels are designed to target two different checkpoints at once.

Take, for instance, the recent breakthrough in targeting PD-L1 and TGF-β. In early clinical trials, this approach has shown promise in notoriously hard-to-treat cancers like colorectal and pancreatic cancer. In the lab, results have been electrifying. Tumors once thought impregnable begin to crumble. Patients with colorectal and pancreatic cancers—diagnoses that once sparked dread in the hearts of oncologists—are showing responses that border on the miraculous.

FS222 is another bispecific antibody, a true double agent in our fight against cancer. This molecule is designed with two different binding sites, allowing it to engage two targets simultaneously. One arm of FS222 latches onto cancer cells, while the other activates killer T cells. FS222 grabs a cancer cell with one molecular hand and a T cell with the other, forcing them into a deadly embrace. This dual action not only marks cancer cells for destruction but also rallies our immune system to join the attack.

Bispecific T cell Engagers, or BiTEs, expand the concept of bispecific antibodies. These synthetic proteins act like molecular matchmakers, bringing cancer cells and T cells into close proximity. One end of the BiTE binds to a specific protein on cancer cells, while the other end binds to T cells. This forced meeting activates the T cells, unleashing their cancer-killing potential. It's as if BiTEs are introducing our immune system's most potent warriors to their mortal enemies, sparking a fierce battle against cancer.

Taking the concept of antibodies a step further, scientists have created **antibody-drug conjugates (ADCs)**. These are like smart bombs in our war against cancer. An ADC consists of a potent anti-cancer drug attached to an antibody. The antibody acts as a guide, leading the drug directly to cancer cells. Once there, the ADC sneaks inside like a Trojan horse, releasing its toxic payload and destroying the cancer from within. This approach minimizes damage to healthy cells, potentially reducing the harsh side effects associated with traditional chemotherapy.

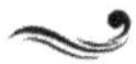

But this is just the beginning of our journey into the complex world of immune regulation. Novel checkpoint targets are unfurling grand possibilities for future cancer treatments. Each new checkpoint we discover, each new combination we try, brings us one step closer to a future where cancer is not a death sentence but a beatable foe. One of the checkpoints at this forefront is **T Cell Immunoglobulin and Mucin domain-containing protein 3,** otherwise known as TIM-3.

TIM-3 is not merely a gatekeeper; it's cunningly strategic. It blocks the entry of immune defenders and actively recruits collaborators to aid in its mission. Picture a bouncer who not only denies access to the good guys but also hands out VIP passes to the tumor's allies—this is TIM-3 in action. By promoting an environment that favors tumor growth, it enhances the cancer's ability to evade detection and destruction.

Moreover, TIM-3 often operates in concert with PD-1. These two are partners in crime, each amplifying the other's effects in suppressing immune responses. When one checkpoint is blocked, the other can compensate, maintaining the tumor's defenses. However, when both TIM-3 and PD-1 are targeted simultaneously, a powerful shift occurs—the tumor's protective barriers begin to crumble.

Early studies focusing on TIM-3 have generated considerable excitement within the research community. By disrupting this dual blockade, scientists are uncovering new avenues for immunotherapy that could significantly enhance anti-tumor responses. This approach holds promise not only for overcoming resistance mechanisms but also for improving outcomes in patients facing some of the most challenging cancers.

TIGIT, or T cell immunoreceptor with Ig and ITIM domains, represents another critical checkpoint protein. This molecular mechanism binds to CD155 and CD112 on tumor cells and antigen-presenting cells, effectively suppressing immune responses. When TIGIT engages with these proteins, it sends inhibitory signals to T cells and natural killer cells, preventing them from mounting an effective attack against cancer cells.

The potential of TIGIT inhibitors lies in their ability to disrupt this suppressive signaling pathway. By blocking TIGIT, researchers aim to remove a significant barrier that prevents immune cells from recognizing and attacking tumors. This approach opens up new possibilities for activating the immune system's natural cancer-fighting capabilities.

Early clinical studies have shown particular promise when TIGIT inhibitors are combined with PD-1 blockers. This dual-targeting strategy addresses multiple immune suppression mechanisms simultaneously, potentially enhancing the overall effectiveness of immunotherapy. By targeting these different checkpoints, researchers hope to overcome the complex defense mechanisms that cancer cells employ to evade immune detection.

Lymphocyte-activation gene 3 (LAG-3) is another important player in this field. We've already learned that when LAG-3 binds to its partners, particularly MHC class II molecules, it can impair a T cell's ability to fight tumors.

Currently, only one LAG-3 inhibitor has reached the U.S. market, and its use is currently restricted to patients with metastatic melanoma. The product must be given alongside a PD-1 inhibitor—a dual-pronged approach that not only reactivates T cells by targeting multiple checkpoints, but can also counter resistance mechanisms that tumors often use to evade treatment. In the future, it may be possible to use LAG-3 targeting to treat a wider range of disease, or use LAG-3 inhibitors alongside other cancer treatments.

Exciting developments in LAG-3 research are pushing the boundaries even further. Bispecific antibodies could maximize immune activation while minimizing the need for multiple drugs. These antibodies simultaneously bind to LAG-3 and PD-1 like a molecular bridge—a strategy that offers unique advantages over traditional single-target antibodies.

The bispecific design allows the antibody to block both checkpoint pathways independently, even if one target is less expressed. Additionally, these antibodies provide a distinct spatial benefit through a phenomenon known as cross-arm avidity.

When the antibody binds one arm to a target like PD-1, it moves very close to the cell surface. Now bound, the second arm is now much closer to its potential target (LAG-3) than it would be if the two arms were approaching independently. This proximity increases the likelihood of the second arm quickly finding and binding to its target. Early studies suggest these antibodies can encourage stronger T cell responses than PD-1 or LAG-3 therapies alone or in combination.

Alternatively, LAG-3 targeting could be achieved through soluble fusion proteins. This approach crafts an entirely new protein using components from LAG-3 immune checkpoints and antibodies. These modified molecules flip LAG-3's usual scripts by converting its inhibitory signals into immune-activating ones. These proteins have already shown potential in combination therapies for late-stage melanoma and breast cancer in clinical trials, paving the way for more breakthroughs in the years to come.

VISTA, or the V-domain Ig suppressor of T cell activation, is another immune checkpoint protein gathering interest. The checkpoint emerges as a master regulator in the immune system's delicate balance. Unlike its counterparts PD-1 and LAG-3, which primarily act as brakes on activated T cells, VISTA plays a more nuanced role. It serves as a gatekeeper of immune quiescence, actively maintaining a state of calm in the immune system even before threats are detected.

VISTA checkpoints act as vigilant sentries, patrolling the borders of our immune system. It doesn't just prevent T cells from attacking; it convinces them there's no reason to be on high alert in the first place. VISTA whispers soothing lullabies to our immune cells, keeping them in a state of tranquility that can be exploited by crafty cancer cells.

But VISTA's influence extends beyond T cells. It acts as a molecular sculptor, shaping the immune landscape to favor tumor growth. VISTA promotes the development of regulatory T cells. It also throws a wrench in the works of dendritic cells, the immune system's intelligence officers, hindering their ability to sound the alarm and activate other immune cells.

In the context of cancer treatment, VISTA becomes particularly intriguing. When other checkpoint inhibitors like PD-1 blockers do their job, VISTA often steps up its game, providing tumors with a backup escape route. It's as if cancer cells have a secret emergency generator, powered by VISTA, that kicks in when their main power supply is cut off.

Targeting VISTA could be a game-changer, especially for patients who don't respond to or develop resistance to other checkpoint inhibitors. It's like cutting off not just the main power to the tumor's fortress, but also disabling its backup systems, leaving cancer cells truly vulnerable to the immune system's assault.

PD-L2, programmed death-ligand 2, another key player in this intricate dance of immune evasion. PD-L2 binds to the same receptor as its more famous cousin PD-L1 (PD-1), but does so with even greater affinity. What's more, PD-L2 is expressed in different patterns than PD-L1. Some tumors that don't respond to PD-1/PD-L1 inhibitors might be using PD-L2 as their primary defense.

Researchers are currently exploring various innovative approaches to address these molecules. For PD-L2, strategies include developing PD-1 inhibitors that block both PD-L1 and PD-L2 binding, creating specific anti-PD-L2 antibodies, incorporating PD-L2 targeting into cancer vaccines, and designing small-molecule drugs to interfere with PD-L2 signaling.

VISTA and PD-L2 stand out as notable targets. Their roles in maintaining immune homeostasis and their potential as backup mechanisms for tumor immune evasion make them promising subjects for future cancer immunotherapies. They join several other inhibitory pathways under investigation that challenge our understanding of the immune system and open up exciting possibilities for treatment.

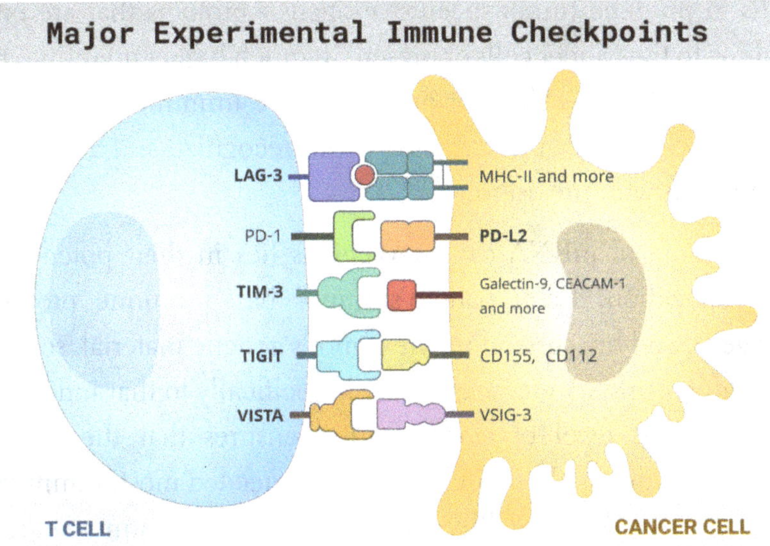

Figure 17. Several, But Not All, Immune Checkpoints Under Investigation. ACCESS HEALTH INTERNATIONAL

In another approach, scientists are harnessing the power of messenger RNA (mRNA) as a formidable weapon against cancer. This innovative technique, which gained global prominence through the development of COVID-19 vaccines, is now being adapted to target and destroy malignant tumors. The underlying principle is simple yet profoundly powerful: by delivering mRNA instructions directly into the body's cells, researchers can teach these cells to produce specific proteins that mount an effective defense against cancer.

In this process, mRNA acts like a stealthy infiltrator, slipping past the defenses of cancer cells and commandeering their resources. Once inside, the mRNA provides the necessary blueprints for the cells to produce tumor-specific antigens—proteins that are either unique to the cancer cells or present in much higher quantities than in normal tissues. This not only alerts the immune system to the presence of cancer but also trains it to recognize and attack these rogue cells with precision.

The beauty of mRNA cancer vaccines lies in their potential for personalization. Each patient’s tumor has a unique profile of antigens, and by sequencing the tumor's genetic material, scientists can design mRNA vaccines tailored specifically to that individual's cancer. This level of customization ensures that the immune response is directed precisely where it is needed most, minimizing collateral damage to healthy cells and enhancing treatment efficacy.

Recent studies have shown that mRNA vaccines can provoke robust immune responses, generating both humoral (antibody-mediated) and cellular (T cell-mediated) immunity. For instance, therapeutic mRNA vaccines have demonstrated stronger immune activation compared to traditional inactivated pathogen or protein-based vaccines. They are capable of stimulating long-lasting immunological memory, which is critical for preventing tumor recurrence after initial treatment.

One particularly promising application is in treating metastatic tumors—those that have spread beyond their original site and are notoriously difficult to eradicate. Research indicates that mRNA vaccines can provoke systemic immune responses capable of targeting these elusive cancer cells throughout the body. In clinical trials, patients receiving personalized mRNA vaccines have shown improvements in their immune response, with some experiencing durable remissions even in advanced stages of cancer.

Alongside refining this technology, scientists are also exploring its integration with other treatment modalities. For example, combining mRNA vaccines with immune checkpoint inhibitors has shown dramatic improvements in patient outcomes. In trials involving high-risk melanoma patients, those receiving a personalized mRNA neoantigen vaccine alongside pembrolizumab—a well-known checkpoint inhibitor—demonstrated significantly better recurrence-free survival compared to those receiving pembrolizumab alone.

The future of mRNA cancer vaccines is bright and filled with promise. With ongoing clinical trials aimed at various malignancies—including pancreatic cancer and glioblastoma—scientists are optimistic about their potential to transform cancer treatment paradigms.

The lessons gleaned from the realm of cancer immunotherapy are proving to be transformative, with implications that extend far beyond oncology. As researchers continue to unravel the complexities of the immune system, we are beginning to see how these insights could reshape the treatment landscape for autoimmune diseases, chronic infections, and even neurodegenerative disorders.

We stand on the precipice of a new era in medicine, where the outdated notion of one-size-fits-all cancer treatment is rapidly becoming a relic of the past. Instead, we are entering a world of precision immunotherapy, where each patient's treatment is meticulously tailored to their unique tumor profile and immune landscape.

Among the most exciting developments in this field is England's National Health Service (NHS) initiative to roll out a groundbreaking seven-minute cancer treatment injection. This innovative approach promises to dramatically reduce treatment times for certain cancer patients. The new method involves administering atezolizumab (Tecentriq) as a subcutaneous injection, which takes only about seven minutes to deliver. This is a remarkable improvement from the traditional intravenous method, which can take anywhere from 30 minutes to an hour.

Atezolizumab is not just any drug; it is an immunotherapy agent that empowers the body's own immune system to seek out and destroy cancer cells. It has been shown to be effective against various cancers, including lung, breast, liver, and bladder cancers. By streamlining its administration, this new approach is expected to enhance patient experience significantly while also freeing up precious time for NHS cancer teams.

The rollout of this innovative treatment method follows its approval by the Medicines and Healthcare products Regulatory Agency (MHRA) and comes at no additional cost to the NHS, thanks to a favorable commercial agreement with Roche, the drug's manufacturer. With approximately 3,600 patients starting atezolizumab treatment annually in England, this transition to a more efficient delivery system could represent a significant leap forward in cancer care.

Progress in the United States may be on the horizon. Biopharmaceutical companies like Merck are undergoing clinical trials that put the concept of injectable checkpoint inhibitors to the test. Recently released data suggests that an injectable form of their PD-1 targeting checkpoint inhibitor, pembrolizumab, can be safely administered alongside chemotherapy for patients with advanced non-small cell lung cancer (NSCL). The method delivers a PD-1 targeting antibody cocktail within two to three minutes and is given every six weeks. So far, this approach delivers comparable results to IV pembrolizumab and chemotherapy.

Looking to the future, it's clear that breakthroughs in cancer treatment are not just possible—they are already unfolding before our eyes. The integration of precision immunotherapy into clinical practice signifies a monumental shift in how we approach cancer care. By harnessing the power of individual patient profiles and leveraging innovative delivery methods like the seven-minute injection, we are moving closer to a future where cancer treatment is more effective and humane.

In this rapidly evolving landscape, every advance brings us one step closer to conquering cancer and improving outcomes for patients. The horizon is bright with promise as we continue our journey into this new era of personalized medicine, where hope and healing go hand in hand.

CHAPTER 9

The Resistance Puzzle

The way cancers develop resistance to treatment is akin to a masterful escape artist, constantly finding new ways to slip free from the chains of therapy. This phenomenon can manifest rapidly, often within weeks of initiating treatment, or emerge stealthily over months or even years. Understanding how cancer cells outsmart treatments is crucial for developing more effective therapies and improving patient outcomes.

One of the most well-known mechanisms of drug resistance involves drug efflux pumps. These are specialized proteins located in the cell membrane. They actively transport anticancer drugs out of the cell before they can exert their therapeutic effects.

A prime example is P-glycoprotein (P-gp), a member of the ATP-binding cassette (ABC) transporter family. When cancer cells overexpress P-gp, they can effectively remove chemotherapy drugs from their interior, reducing drug concentrations to subtherapeutic levels. This means that even when a patient receives a full dose of medication, the cancer cells are able to evade its effects by simply pushing it out.

Research has shown that P-gp and other efflux pumps like ABCC1, multidrug resistance-associated protein 1, and ABCG2, breast cancer resistance protein, can confer multidrug resistance by expelling a wide range of chemotherapeutic agents, including anthracyclines and taxanes.

Another cunning strategy employed by cancer cells involves altering the very targets that drugs are designed to attack. For instance, if a chemotherapy drug works by binding to a specific protein on the cancer cell, mutations in that protein can prevent the drug from binding effectively. This phenomenon has been observed in cancers such as lung cancer, where mutations in the epidermal growth factor receptor (EGFR) gene can render targeted therapies ineffective. Such mutations allow cancer cells to continue proliferating despite treatment efforts.

Cancer cells are remarkably adaptable and can change their behavior in response to treatment pressures. For example, when exposed to chemotherapy, some cells may enter a state of dormancy, avoiding division and thus evading the effects of drugs that target rapidly dividing cells. Once treatment ceases or is lessened, these dormant cells can reactivate and repopulate the tumor, leading to relapse.

As we have seen, the tumor microenvironment also plays a critical role in resistance. Cancer cells exist within a complex ecosystem consisting of surrounding stromal cells, immune cells, and extracellular matrix components that can influence their behavior.

Factors released by these surrounding cells can promote survival pathways in cancer cells, making them more resistant to therapies. For instance, certain cytokines produced by immune cells can enhance survival signals in tumor cells, allowing them to withstand the effects of chemotherapy.

Moreover, tumors are not composed of identical cells; instead, they exhibit significant genetic diversity known as heterogeneity. This means that within a single tumor, some cancer cells may be sensitive to treatment while others are resistant due to different genetic mutations or expression patterns. As treatment progresses, resistant clones may survive and proliferate, leading to a more aggressive disease that is harder to treat.

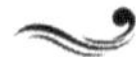

Researchers are actively exploring various strategies to combat the persistent challenges posed by cancer treatment resistance, with combination therapies emerging as a pivotal approach. This strategy involves the use of multiple drugs that operate through different mechanisms of action, either simultaneously or sequentially, to enhance therapeutic efficacy and reduce the likelihood that cancer cells will develop resistance.

The rationale for combination therapies is grounded in the complex biology of cancer. Tumors are not homogeneous; they consist of diverse populations of cells that can exhibit varying responses to treatment due to genetic mutations, epigenetic modifications, and differences in microenvironmental factors. This intra-tumor heterogeneity means that while some cancer cells may be sensitive to a particular drug, others may possess mutations or expression patterns that confer resistance.

A common approach in cancer treatment is to combine chemotherapy with targeted therapy or immunotherapy. Chemotherapy drugs typically work by damaging the DNA of rapidly dividing cells, while targeted therapies focus on specific molecular targets involved in cancer growth and survival. When used together, these therapies can create a multi-faceted attack on the tumor, effectively addressing its complexity.

Research has shown that such pairings can lead to synergistic effects, where the combined impact of the drugs is greater than the sum of their individual effects. This synergy enhances overall treatment efficacy and can potentially lead to better patient outcomes. For instance, combining a chemotherapeutic agent like doxorubicin with a targeted agent such as trastuzumab, which specifically targets HER2-positive breast cancer, has been shown to enhance cell death more effectively than either drug alone.

Studies have demonstrated that this combination not only improves therapeutic outcomes but also reduces the risk of resistance development by simultaneously attacking multiple pathways within the cancer cells. By leveraging these synergistic interactions, combination therapies represent a powerful strategy in the fight against cancer, offering hope for improved effectiveness and durability of treatment responses.

Different drugs can target distinct signaling pathways involved in tumor growth and survival. For example, combining an angiogenesis inhibitor, which prevents tumor blood vessel formation, with a cytotoxic agent can simultaneously starve the tumor of nutrients while directly killing cancer cells. This dual approach has been shown to improve treatment responses in various cancers

The clinical application of combination therapies has yielded promising results across various cancer types. For instance, in metastatic breast cancer, combining chemotherapy with targeted agents has led to improved progression-free survival rates compared to monotherapy approaches. Similarly, in pancreatic cancer, administering gemcitabine with other agents has demonstrated enhanced efficacy and reduced resistance development.

Moreover, ongoing research is focused on optimizing the sequencing and timing of drug administration within combination regimens. This strategic approach aims to maximize therapeutic benefits while minimizing toxicity to normal tissues. For example, administering a targeted therapy before chemotherapy may sensitize cancer cells to subsequent treatments by disrupting their survival pathways

Innovations such as restrictive combinations, which strategically select drugs based on their differential effects on normal versus cancerous cells, are being explored as potential methods to enhance therapeutic indices while reducing side effects. Additionally, advances in artificial intelligence and machine learning are being used to identify novel drug combinations that might not be immediately apparent through conventionall research methods.

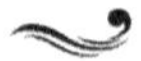

Another promising concept in the fight against cancer resistance is the use of Proteolysis-Targeting Chimeras or PROTACs. PROTACs represent a paradigm shift in how we approach cancer treatment. These ingenious molecules act as molecular bounty hunters, tagging cancer-causing proteins for destruction by the cell's own protein degradation machinery. Imagine a scenario where we can turn cancer's cellular recycling system against itself, transforming it into a precision demolition team that selectively eliminates the very proteins driving tumor growth.

The beauty of PROTACs lies in their ability to overcome resistance mechanisms that have long frustrated oncologists. In cases where cancer cells stubbornly overproduce certain proteins or develop mutations that render traditional drugs ineffective, PROTACs offer a fresh approach. By targeting these problematic proteins for complete degradation, rather than merely inhibiting their function, PROTACs can potentially sidestep many of the resistance mechanisms that have stymied previous treatments.

Recent studies have shown promising results. For instance, researchers have developed PROTACs that can effectively degrade mutant forms of the androgen receptor in prostate cancer cells that have become resistant to standard hormone therapies. This breakthrough offers new hope for patients with advanced prostate cancer who have exhausted other treatment options.

PROTACs are bifunctional, meaning they consist of two distinct ligands connected by a linker: one ligand binds to the target protein, while the other recruits an E3 ubiquitin ligase. This unique design allows PROTACs to effectively bring the target protein into close proximity with the E3 ligase, facilitating the addition of ubiquitin molecules. Once tagged with ubiquitin, the target protein is recognized by the proteasome for degradation.

The ability of PROTACs to induce targeted protein degradation offers a significant advantage in cases where resistance arises due to protein overexpression or mutations. For instance, when cancer cells adapt to therapies by producing excess amounts of a specific protein that drives their growth, traditional inhibitors may become ineffective. However, PROTACs can bypass this issue by degrading the problematic protein entirely rather than merely inhibiting its function. This approach not only reduces the levels of oncoproteins but also helps prevent the emergence of resistant cell populations.

Moreover, PROTACs have shown promise in targeting traditionally "undruggable" proteins— those that lack suitable binding sites for conventional small-molecule inhibitors. This includes challenging targets like transcription factors and certain kinases that play critical roles in tumor progression. By exploiting the ubiquitin-proteasome system, PROTACs can effectively degrade these difficult targets, opening new avenues for treatment where traditional therapies have failed.

Recent advances in PROTAC technology have led to several candidates entering clinical trials, demonstrating their potential as effective anticancer agents. For example, ARV-110 targets the androgen receptor in prostate cancer, while ARV-471 focuses on the estrogen receptor in breast cancer. These trials not only highlight the versatility of PROTACs but also their capacity to overcome resistance mechanisms associated with mutations and overexpression.

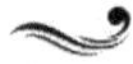

Furthermore, In the realm of cancer research, sometimes old players reveal new tricks. Vitamin D, long known for its role in bone health, has emerged as a potential ally in the fight against cancer. Recent studies have shed light on vitamin D's ability to enhance antitumor immune responses, offering a new perspective on this familiar nutrient..

Emerging research has revealed that vitamin D may play a crucial role in enhancing our body's natural defenses against cancer. This humble vitamin appears to have a remarkable ability to modulate the immune system, potentially boosting its capacity to recognize and attack cancer cells. Studies have shown that vitamin D can influence various immune cells, including T cells and dendritic cells, which act as the commanders and foot soldiers in our body's war against tumors.

Moreover, vitamin D seems to have direct effects on cancer cells themselves, potentially putting the brakes on their growth and spread. Some studies have suggested that maintaining adequate vitamin D levels may be associated with better outcomes in certain cancer types, though researchers caution that more investigation is needed to fully understand these relationships.

Amidst the complex interplay between nutrition, immunity, and cancer, vitamin D stands out as a promising area of investigation. Its potential to enhance antitumor responses, coupled with its relative safety and accessibility, makes it an intriguing subject for further study in the context of cancer treatment and prevention.

The journey to overcome cancer resistance is far from over, but each discovery brings us closer to more effective and durable treatments. By combining innovative approaches like PROTACs with insights into the role of nutrients like vitamin D, we edge ever closer to turning the tide in our favor in the battle against cancer. The war may be long and arduous, but with each breakthrough, we arm ourselves with new weapons and strategies, inching closer to a future where cancer's ability to resist our treatments becomes a relic of the past.

CHAPTER 10

From Cancer to Chronic Conditions

When researchers first targeted checkpoint proteins to fight cancer, they couldn't have predicted how far-reaching their discovery would become. These molecular switches could become central players in diseases where immune regulation goes awry. Scientists are repurposing knowledge of checkpoint pathways to tackle challenges such as calming the self-destructive immune responses in rheumatoid arthritis, protecting brain cells in Alzheimer's disease, and reinvigorating immune cells exhausted by chronic viral infections.

In cancer treatment, we've learned to silence checkpoint proteins, allowing the immune system to play at full volume against tumor cells. But this same understanding could be turned on its head: in autoimmune diseases, where the immune orchestra plays too loudly, we might amplify these checkpoint signals to soften the response. In neurodegenerative conditions, we could fine-tune them to protect vulnerable brain cells. And in chronic viral infections, we might adjust their activity to help exhausted immune cells regain their strength. It's a striking reminder that in science, breakthrough insights often echo into unexpected territories, creating new possibilities for treating previously intractable diseases.

In autoimmune diseases like rheumatoid arthritis, lupus, and type 1 diabetes, the immune system mistakenly attacks the body's tissues. Researchers discovered early on that checkpoint proteins are crucial in preventing these autoimmune attacks. Now, they are exploring how to use PD-1's natural braking ability to dial these autoresponses back.

Recent research has revealed a fascinating secret about PD-1: it works best in pairs. Scientists have discovered that when two PD-1 proteins form a "dimer," they become much more effective at suppressing immune cell activity. This discovery has opened up an exciting new avenue for autoimmune disease treatment. Instead of blocking PD-1 like in cancer therapy, researchers are now working on drugs that encourage PD-1 proteins to pair up. It's like giving the immune system's brake pedal an extra boost.

These new drugs, called PD-1 agonists, are designed to stimulate PD-1 activity. Early clinical trials show promising results for rheumatoid arthritis, lupus, and type 1 diabetes. By enhancing PD-1's natural braking ability, these treatments aim to gently calm overactive immune responses without completely shutting down the immune system.

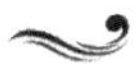

The role of inflammation in neurodegenerative diseases such as Alzheimer's and Parkinson's is becoming increasingly clear. Could checkpoint inhibitors, with their potential to modulate immune responses, offer a new and intriguing avenue for treatment?

In neurodegenerative diseases, the delicate balance in the brain's ecosystem is disrupted, and inflammation becomes a double-edged sword: On one hand, some inflammation is necessary for the brain's natural cleaning and repair processes. Conversely, chronic, unchecked inflammation can damage healthy brain cells and accelerate disease progression.

Checkpoint inhibitors have the potential to offer several benefits by fine-tuning the immune response. These drugs could help reduce harmful inflammation by modulating immune activity, which may be beneficial in dampening chronic inflammation that contributes to brain cell damage. A controlled immune response could also enhance the brain's ability to clear out toxic protein aggregates, such as amyloid plaques in Alzheimer's, without causing additional harm.

Moreover, checkpoint inhibitors help protect healthy neurons by creating a more balanced immune environment, shielding them from inflammatory damage. Some researchers also speculate that a carefully modulated immune response could support the brain's natural repair mechanisms, promoting repair. The possibilities are undoubtedly worth exploring.

Although research is still in its early stages, the ability to fine-tune immune responses using PD-1 modulators could potentially help in three ways: reducing harmful inflammation in the brain, promoting the clearance of toxic protein aggregates, and supporting the survival of healthy neurons.

Current treatments for autoimmune diseases often involve broad immunosuppression, which can leave patients vulnerable to infections. PD-1 agonists offer the potential for a more targeted approach. They work by focusing on a specific immune checkpoint, potentially causing fewer side effects than general immunosuppressants. These drugs enhance a natural process in the body, leading to a more balanced immune response. Early research suggests that PD-1 agonists might be able to act more specifically in areas of inflammation rather than suppressing the entire immune system.

From autoimmune diseases to neurodegenerative disorders, checkpoint inhibitors represent a promising new medical frontier. By learning to fine-tune our immune system's natural brakes and accelerators, we may one day have powerful new tools to treat a wide range of chronic conditions.

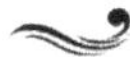

Our immune system faces a formidable challenge in chronic viral infections, such as HIV and hepatitis C. Over time, the constant battle against these persistent invaders can leave our T cells—the frontline soldiers of our adaptive immune response—exhausted, ineffective, and unable to muster the strength for one more charge against the enemy.

PD-1, our now-familiar immune checkpoint protein, is at the heart of this exhaustion. In chronic infections, PD-1 becomes overexpressed on T cells, acting like a constant brake that prevents them from mounting an adequate response. It's as if our immune system, in an attempt to avoid collateral damage from an overzealous response, inadvertently allows the virus to gain the upper hand.

But what if we could rejuvenate these tired T cells?

This is where the exciting potential of PD-1 modulation comes into play. Researchers are exploring ways to adjust PD-1 activity to strike a delicate balance carefully. The goal is to reinvigorate exhausted T cells just enough to effectively combat the virus without unleashing an uncontrolled immune response that could harm healthy tissues. Physicians will need to closely monitor patients for immune-related adverse effects and prescribe immunosuppressants as soon as a new infection develops or the existing infection worsens. Early studies have shown promising results, with carefully timed and dosed PD-1 blockade leading to improved viral control and T cell function in chronic infections.

The recent discovery of PD-1's ability to form dimers—pairs of PD-1 molecules working in tandem—has added an intriguing new dimension to this research. This finding is like uncovering a secret weapon in our immune arsenal that could be wielded differently depending on the battle.

In the fight against cancer, future drugs might aim to break apart these PD-1 dimers, potentially making our current immunotherapies even more potent. It's like finding a way to turn off the enemy's shields, allowing our immune system to launch a more effective assault on tumor cells.

Conversely, when it comes to taming autoimmune diseases, the strategy flips. Here, treatments could focus on encouraging PD-1 dimers to form, strengthening the immune system's natural brakes. This approach is akin to reinforcing the walls that keep an overzealous immune response in check, offering relief to those suffering from conditions where the body attacks itself.

Perhaps most excitingly, this new understanding of PD-1's transmembrane domain—the part of the protein that spans the cell membrane—opens up new avenues for drug development. It's as if we've discovered a new lock, and now we can craft keys that fit it perfectly, whether to open or secure it as needed.

However, as with all medical frontiers, challenges abound. The immune system is an intricate ballet of checks and balances, and tinkering with it requires the utmost precision. Achieving the right level of immune modulation for each condition will be crucial. Too much activation could lead to harmful inflammation or autoimmune-like side effects. At the same time, too little might render the treatment ineffective.

Safety concerns loom large, particularly when considering long-term use of these therapies. Our immune system is our body's guardian, and altering its function, even with the best intentions, could have unforeseen consequences. Vigilant monitoring for unexpected side effects will be essential as these treatments move from the lab to the clinic.

Moreover, the incredible diversity of human immune systems means that a one-size-fits-all approach is unlikely to succeed. Just as each person's fingerprint is unique, so is their immune signature. Developing personalized treatment strategies that account for individual variations in immune function will be a complex but necessary challenge.

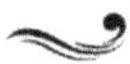

The unfurling of one field of medicine could give way to another. Checkpoint research may have blossomed in the context of cancer, but it has the potential to stretch far and wide, from cancer to autoimmune diseases, from persistent viral infections to neurodegenerative disorders. While the road ahead is long and winding, there desire to transform lives makes every step of the journey worthwhile. Unraveling the complexities of our immune system brings us closer to a future where some of our most challenging chronic conditions may finally meet their match.

A Final Word

As we close this journey through the science of checkpoint inhibitors, we return to a simple truth: cancers are not just medical conditions—they are a deeply human experience. From Richard Metz's remarkable story to the countless others whose lives have been touched by this disease, we've seen how checkpoint inhibitors have rewritten what's possible in cancer care. These treatments don't just target tumors; they restore hope, return precious time, and redefine what it means to live with cancer.

And yet, another truth rings true: there is no such thing as a 'perfect' cancer treatment. Every therapeutic comes with its own boons and pitfalls—and checkpoint inhibitors are no exception. These drugs are without question a breakthrough, a testament to the power of immunotherapy to meet cancer with our body's own defenses, especially when options are scarce. However, while checkpoint inhibitors show great promise against some cancers, their reach is uneven. Each patient and tumor type brings unique challenges, and researchers are steadily working to refine the therapy—understanding who will benefit most, maximizing the impact, and extending the life of each response.

But there is hope on the horizon. If cancer is an elusive target, science is learning to shift with it. Innovative technologies and new insights into immunity are changing cancer care and slowly uncovering the untapped potential of these treatments. Each breakthrough offers a clearer view of cancer's vulnerabilities, illuminating a path forward.

The dream we chase is lasting remission, a return to life before illness, the assurance that even advanced cancer will not return. While no single therapy has yet mastered this task, the quantity and quality of our treatment arsenal grows stronger every year. Long-term remissions suggest we're tantalizingly close to this goal, each approach working from different angles to anticipate cancer's moves. And with checkpoint inhibitors, we have a powerful ally—one that can enhance both traditional therapies and new innovations, delivering results we previously couldn't imagine.

Checkpoint inhibitors are not a cure to cancer, but they are a vital step in realizing this dream. They serve as a marker of how far we've come in cancer treatment and as a beacon for what lies ahead. And though the journey continues, with every new stride, the weight of the word 'cancer' grows a little lighter.

References

This book's referencing is organized by chapter to facilitate a more streamlined and accessible reading experience. Each chapter includes its own set of references, allowing readers to easily locate sources relevant to the specific content discussed within that section. Readers are encouraged to consult the references at the end of each chapter to further explore the themes and concepts discussed.

Introduction

1. Richard: Melanoma Survivor. Yale Medicine. https://www.yalemedicine.org/survivor-stories/richard-skin-cancer-survivor
2. Survivor Perspective: Brain Metastasis. Yale Medicine. Published August 4, 2013. Accessed November 12, 2024. https://www.yalemedicine.org/podcasts/cancer-answers-survivor-perspective-brain-metasasis-august-4-2013
3. Internò V, Maria Chiara Sergi, Maria Elvira Metta, et al. Melanoma Brain Metastases: A Retrospective Analysis of Prognostic Factors and Efficacy of Multimodal Therapies. *Cancers.* 2023;15(5):1542-1542. doi:https://doi.org/10.3390/cancers15051542

Chapter 1

1. Faguet GB. A brief history of cancer: Age-old milestones underlying our current knowledge database. *International*

Journal of Cancer. 2014;136(9):2022-2036. doi:https://doi.org/10.1002/ijc.29134

2. Mendiratta G, Ke E, Aziz M, Liarakos D, Tong M, Stites EC. Cancer gene mutation frequencies for the U.S. population. *Nature Communications.* 2021;12(1):5961. doi:https://doi.org/10.1038/s41467-021-26213-y

3. Seyfried TN, Huysentruyt LC. On the origin of cancer metastasis. *Critical Reviews in Oncogenesis.* 2013;18(1-2):43-73. doi:https://doi.org/10.1615/critrevoncog.v18.i1-2.40

4. Birch JM, Blair V. The epidemiology of infant cancers. *The British Journal of Cancer Supplement.* 1992;18:S2. Accessed November 12, 2024. https://pmc.ncbi.nlm.nih.gov/articles/PMC2149659/

5. Laconi E, Marongiu F, DeGregori J. Cancer as a disease of old age: changing mutational and microenvironmental landscapes. *British Journal of Cancer.* 2020;122(7):943-952. doi:https://doi.org/10.1038/s41416-019-0721-1

6. National Cancer Institute. Cancer Statistics. National Cancer Institute. Published May 9, 2024. https://www.cancer.gov/about-cancer/understanding/statistics

7. National Cancer Institute. Age and Cancer Risk. National Cancer Institute. Published March 5, 2021. https://www.cancer.gov/about-cancer/causes-prevention/risk/age

8. Caplan Z. U.S. older population grew from 2010 to 2020 at fastest rate since 1880 to 1890. United States Census Bureau. Published May 25, 2023. https://www.census.gov/library/stories/2023/05/2020-census-united-states-older-population-grew.html

9. Curtin S, Tejada-Vera B, Bastian B. *National Vital Statistics Reports Deaths: Leading Causes for 2020.*; 2023. https://www.cdc.gov/nchs/data/nvsr/nvsr72/nvsr72-13.pdf

10. Tonorezos E, Devasia T, Mariotto AB, et al. Prevalence of cancer survivors in the United States. *JNCI Journal of the National Cancer Institute*. Published online July 13, 2024. doi:https://doi.org/10.1093/jnci/djae135

11. Cui J, Ding Rong-mei, Liu H, Ma M, Zuo RC, Liu X. Trends in the incidence and survival of cancer in individuals aged 55 years and older in the United States, 1975–2019. *BMC Public Health.* 2024;24(1). doi:https://doi.org/10.1186/s12889-023-17571-x

12. Kort EJ, Paneth N, Vande GF. The Decline in U.S. Cancer Mortality in People Born since 1925. 2009;69(16):6500-6505. doi:https://doi.org/10.1158/0008-5472.can-09-0357

13. Siegel RL, Miller KD, Fuchs HE, Jemal A. Cancer statistics, 2022. *CA: A Cancer Journal for Clinicians.* 2022;72(1):7-33. doi:https://doi.org/10.3322/caac.21708

14. Cancer patients cured a decade after gene therapy, doctors say. NBC News. https://www.nbcnews.com/health/cancer/cancer-patients-cured-decade-gene-therapy-doctors-say-rcna14630

Chapter 2

1. Science Talk - "Immunotherapy is keeping me alive" - John's story - The Institute of Cancer Research, London. Icr.ac.uk. Published 2023. Accessed November 12, 2024. https://www.icr.ac.uk/blogs/science-talk/page-details/immunotherapy-is-keeping-me-alive---john-s-story
2. Only 14% of Cancers Are Detected Through a Preventive Screening Test. https://www.norc.org/content/dam/norc-org/pdfs/State-Specific%20PCDSs%20chart%201213.pdf
3. Sharma I, Sharma A, Tomer R, Negi N, Ranbir Chander Sobti. History, Evolution, Milestones in Cancer Research and Treatment. Published online January 1, 2023:1-29. doi:https://doi.org/10.1007/978-981-99-2196-6_2-1
4. Baskar R, Lee KA, Yeo R, Yeoh KW. Cancer and Radiation Therapy: Current Advances and Future Directions. *International Journal of Medical Sciences*. 2012;9(3):193-199. doi:https://doi.org/10.7150/ijms.3635
5. Majeed H, Gupta V. Adverse Effects Of Radiation Therapy. PubMed. Published August 14, 2023. https://www.ncbi.nlm.nih.gov/books/NBK563259/
6. Rockwell S. The Life and Legacy of Marie Curie. https://europepmc.org/backend/ptpmcrender.fcgi?accid=PMC2582731&blobtype=pdf
7. Faguet GB. A brief history of cancer: Age-old milestones underlying our current knowledge database. *International Journal of Cancer*. 2014;136(9):2022-2036. doi:https://doi.org/10.1002/ijc.29134

8. x.com. X (formerly Twitter). Published 2024. Accessed November 12, 2024. https://x.com/John_Dabell/status/1430152018895724546

9. Haseltine W. CAR T: A New Cure for Cancer, Autoimmune and Inherited Disease: Haseltine, William A, Thomas, Amara: 9798989082346: Amazon.com: Books. Amazon.com. Published 2024. Accessed November 12, 2024. https://www.amazon.com/CAR-Cancer-Autoimmune-Inherited-Disease/dp/B0CMH7MKPL

10. Falzone L, Salomone S, Libra M. Evolution of Cancer Pharmacological Treatments at the Turn of the Third Millennium. *Frontiers in Pharmacology.* 2018;9(1300). doi:https://doi.org/10.3389/fphar.2018.01300

Chapter 3

1. Dobosz P, Dzieciątkowski T. The Intriguing History of Cancer Immunotherapy. *Frontiers in Immunology.* 2019;10(2965). doi:https://doi.org/10.3389/fimmu.2019.02965

2. McCarthy EF. The toxins of William B. Coley and the treatment of bone and soft-tissue sarcomas. *The Iowa orthopaedic journal.* 2006;26:154-158. https://www.ncbi.nlm.nih.gov/pmc/articles/PMC1888599/

3. Zhang Y, Zhang Z. The history and advances in cancer immunotherapy: understanding the characteristics of tumor-infiltrating immune cells and their therapeutic implications. *Cellular & Molecular Immunology.*

2020;17(8):1-15. doi:https://doi.org/10.1038/s41423-020-0488-6

4. Steinman RM, Cohn ZA. IDENTIFICATION OF A NOVEL CELL TYPE IN PERIPHERAL LYMPHOID ORGANS OF MICE. *Journal of Experimental Medicine.* 1973;137(5):1142-1162. doi:https://doi.org/10.1084/jem.137.5.1142
5. Kiessling R, Klein E, Pross H, Wigzell H. „Natural" killer cells in the mouse. II. Cytotoxic cells with specificity for mouse Moloney leukemia cells. Characteristics of the killer cell. *European Journal of Immunology.* 1975;5(2):117-121. doi:https://doi.org/10.1002/eji.1830050209
6. Brunet JF, Denizot F, Luciani MF, et al. A new member of the immunoglobulin superfamily—CTLA-4. *Nature.* 1987;328(6127):267-270. doi:https://doi.org/10.1038/328267a0
7. Waterhouse P, Penninger JM, Timms E, et al. Lymphoproliferative Disorders with Early Lethality in Mice Deficient in Ctla-4. *Science.* 1995;270(5238):985-988. doi:https://doi.org/10.1126/science.270.5238.985
8. Walunas TL, Lenschow DJ, Bakker CY, Green JM, Thompson CB, Bluestone JA. CTLA-4 can function as a negative regulator of T cell activation. Published 1994. https://www.cell.com/immunity/abstract/1074-7613(94)90071-X
9. Tivol EA, Borriello F, Schweitzer ANicola, Lynch WP, Bluestone JA, Sharpe AH. Loss of CTLA-4 leads to massive lymphoproliferation and fatal multiorgan tissue

destruction, revealing a critical negative regulatory role of CTLA-4. Published 1995. https://www.sciencedirect.com/science/article/pii/1074761395901256

10. Krummel MF, Allison JP. CD28 and CTLA-4 have opposing effects on the response of T cells to stimulation. *The Journal of Experimental Medicine.* 1995;182(2):459-465. doi:https://doi.org/10.1084/jem.182.2.459

11. Leach DR, Krummel MF, Allison JP. Enhancement of Antitumor Immunity by CTLA-4 Blockade. *Science.* 1996;271(5256):1734-1736. doi:https://doi.org/10.1126/science.271.5256.1734

12. National Inventors Hall of Fame - NIHF. Rebel Scientist: The James Allison Story. YouTube. Published May 4, 2024. Accessed November 12, 2024. https://www.youtube.com/watch?v=oQlKJBS9CaQ

13. The Nobel Prize in Physiology or Medicine 2018. NobelPrize.org. Published 2024. Accessed November 12, 2024. https://www.nobelprize.org/prizes/medicine/2018/allison/159229-james-allison-interview-transcript/

14. Hodi FS, Mihm MC, Soiffer RJ, et al. Biologic activity of cytotoxic T lymphocyte-associated antigen 4 antibody blockade in previously vaccinated metastatic melanoma and ovarian carcinoma patients. *Proceedings of the National Academy of Sciences of the United States of America.* 2003;100(8):4712-4717. doi:https://doi.org/10.1073/pnas.0830997100

15. Hodi FS, O'Day SJ, McDermott DF, et al. Improved Survival with Ipilimumab in Patients with Metastatic Melanoma. *New England Journal of Medicine*. 2010;363(8):711-723.

16. Robert C, Thomas L, Bondarenko I, et al. Ipilimumab plus Dacarbazine for Previously Untreated Metastatic Melanoma. *New England Journal of Medicine*. 2011;364(26):2517-2526. doi:https://doi.org/10.1056/nejmoa1104621

17. *HIGHLIGHTS of PRESCRIBING INFORMATION*. https://www.accessdata.fda.gov/drugsatfda_docs/label/2020/125377s115lbl.pdf

18. Ishida Y, Agata Y, Shibahara K, Honjo T. Induced expression of PD-1, a novel member of the immunoglobulin gene superfamily, upon programmed cell death. *The EMBO Journal*. 1992;11(11):3887-3895. doi:https://doi.org/10.1002/j.1460-2075.1992.tb05481.x

19. Ishida Y. PD-1: Its Discovery, Involvement in Cancer Immunotherapy, and Beyond. *Cells*. 2020;9(6):1376. doi:https://doi.org/10.3390/cells9061376

20. Smith C, Williams GT, Kingston R, Jenkinson EJ, Owen J. Antibodies to CD3/T-cell receptor complex induce death by apoptosis in immature T cells in thymic cultures. 1989;337(6203):181-184. doi:https://doi.org/10.1038/337181a0

21. The Nobel Prize in Physiology or Medicine 2018. NobelPrize.org.

https://www.nobelprize.org/prizes/medicine/2018/honjo/159695-tasuku-honjo-interview-transcript/

22. Nishimura H, Nose M, Hiai H, Minato N, Honjo T. Development of Lupus-like Autoimmune Diseases by Disruption of the PD-1 Gene Encoding an ITIM Motif-Carrying Immunoreceptor. *Immunity*. 1999;11(2):141-151. doi:https://doi.org/10.1016/s1074-7613(00)80089-8

23. Nishimura H. Autoimmune Dilated Cardiomyopathy in PD-1 Receptor-Deficient Mice. *Science*. 2001;291(5502):319-322. doi:https://doi.org/10.1126/science.291.5502.319

24. Wang J, Yoshida T, Nakaki F, Hiai H, Okazaki T, Honjo T. Establishment of NOD-Pdcd1-/- mice as an efficient animal model of type I diabetes. *Proceedings of the National Academy of Sciences*. 2005;102(33):11823-11828. doi:https://doi.org/10.1073/pnas.0505497102

25. Dong H, Zhu G, Tamada K, Chen L. B7-H1, a third member of the B7 family, co-stimulates T-cell proliferation and interleukin-10 secretion. *Nature Medicine*. 1999;5(12):1365-1369. doi:https://doi.org/10.1038/70932

26. Freeman GJ, Long AJ, Iwai Y, et al. Engagement of the Pd-1 Immunoinhibitory Receptor by a Novel B7 Family Member Leads to Negative Regulation of Lymphocyte Activation. *The Journal of Experimental Medicine*. 2000;192(7):1027-1034. doi:https://doi.org/10.1084/jem.192.7.1027

27. Latchman Y, Wood CR, Chernova T, et al. PD-L2 is a second ligand for PD-1 and inhibits T cell activation.

Nature Immunology. 2001;2(3):261-268. doi:https://doi.org/10.1038/85330

28. Liang Spencer C, Greenwald Rebecca J, Latchman Yvette E, et al. PD-L1 and PD-L2 have distinct roles in regulating host immunity to cutaneous leishmaniasis. *European Journal of Immunology*. 2006;36(1):58-64. doi:https://doi.org/10.1002/eji.200535458

29. Latchman YE, Liang SC, Wu Y, et al. PD-L1-deficient mice show that PD-L1 on T cells, antigen-presenting cells, and host tissues negatively regulates T cells. *Proceedings of the National Academy of Sciences*. 2004;101(29):10691-10696. doi:https://doi.org/10.1073/pnas.0307252101

30. Iwai Y, Ishida M, Tanaka Y, Okazaki T, Honjo T, Minato N. Involvement of PD-L1 on tumor cells in the escape from host immune system and tumor immunotherapy by PD-L1 blockade. *Proceedings of the National Academy of Sciences*. 2002;99(19):12293-12297. doi:https://doi.org/10.1073/pnas.192461099

31. Phase I Study of Single-Agent Anti–Programmed Death-1 (MDX-1106) in Refractory Solid Tumors: Safety, Clinical Activity, Pharmacodynamics, and Immunologic Correlates | Journal of Clinical Oncology. Journal of Clinical Oncology. Published 2014. Accessed November 12, 2024. https://ascopubs.org/doi/10.1200/JCO.2009.26.7609

32. *CENTER for DRUG EVALUATION and RESEARCH Approval Package For.* https://www.accessdata.fda.gov/drugsatfda_docs/nda/2014/125514Orig1s000Approv.pdf

33. Myers B. *CENTER for DRUG EVALUATION and RESEARCH Approval Package For: APPLICATION NUMBER: 125554Orig1s000 Trade Name: Opdivo Generic Name: Nivolumab Sponsor: Indications.*; 2014. https://www.accessdata.fda.gov/drugsatfda_docs/nda/2014/125554Orig1s000Approv.pdf

34. Bernard N. Origin of immune checkpoint inhibitors. *Nature Research.* Published online December 6, 2022. doi:https://doi.org/10.1038/d42859-022-00046-1

35. Vogel G. Cancer immunotherapy pioneers win medicine Nobel. *Science.* Published online October 1, 2018. doi:https://doi.org/10.1126/science.aav5901

Chapter 4

1. Dean L. Blood Groups and Red Cell Antigens. National Library of Medicine. Published 2005. https://www.ncbi.nlm.nih.gov/books/NBK2263/

2. Lythe G, Callard RE, Hoare RL, Molina-París C. How many TCR clonotypes does a body maintain? *Journal of Theoretical Biology.* 2016;389:214-224. doi:https://doi.org/10.1016/j.jtbi.2015.10.016

3. Chen L, Flies DB. Molecular mechanisms of T cell co-stimulation and co-inhibition. *Nature Reviews Immunology.* 2013;13(4):227-242. doi:https://doi.org/10.1038/nri3405

4. Frauwirth KA, Thompson CB. Activation and inhibition of lymphocytes by costimulation. *The Journal of Clinical*

Investigation. 2002;109(3):295-299. doi:https://doi.org/10.1172/JCI14941

5. Md. Munnaf Hossen, Ma Y, Yin Z, et al. Current understanding of CTLA-4: from mechanism to autoimmune diseases. *Frontiers in Immunology*. 2023;14. doi:https://doi.org/10.3389/fimmu.2023.1198365
6. Buchbinder E, Desai A. February 2016 - Volume 39 - Issue 1 : American Journal of Clinical Oncology. journals.lww.com. Published February 2016. https://journals.lww.com/amjclinicaloncology/Fulltext/2016/02000/CTLA_4_and_PD_1_Pathways__Similarities
7. Wu X, Gu Z, Chen Y, et al. Application of PD-1 Blockade in Cancer Immunotherapy. *Computational and structural biotechnology journal*. 2019;17:661-674. doi:https://doi.org/10.1016/j.csbj.2019.03.006

Chapter 5

1. Fecher LA, Agarwala SS, Hodi FS, Weber JS. Ipilimumab and Its Toxicities: A Multidisciplinary Approach. *The Oncologist*. 2013;18(6):733-743. doi:https://doi.org/10.1634/theoncologist.2012-0483
2. To SY, Lee CH, Chen YH, et al. Psoriasis Risk With Immune Checkpoint Inhibitors. *JAMA Dermatology*. Published online November 6, 2024. doi:https://doi.org/10.1001/jamadermatol.2024.4129
3. Kotwal A, Haddox C, Block M, Kudva YC. Immune checkpoint inhibitors: an emerging cause of insulin-dependent diabetes. *BMJ Open Diabetes Research & Care*.

2019;7(1):e000591. doi:https://doi.org/10.1136/bmjdrc-2018-000591

4. Cancer History Project. Melanoma survivor Sharon Belvin meets Dr. Jim Allison for the first time. Cancer History Project. Published 2023. Accessed November 21, 2024. https://cancerhistoryproject.com/article/melanoma-survivor-sharon-belvin-meets-dr-jim-allison-for-the-first-time/
5. *CENTER for DRUG EVALUATION and RESEARCH Approval Package For.* https://www.accessdata.fda.gov/drugsatfda_docs/nda/2014/125514Orig1s000Approv.pdf
6. Myers B. *CENTER for DRUG EVALUATION and RESEARCH Approval Package For: APPLICATION NUMBER: 125554Orig1s000 Trade Name: Opdivo Generic Name: Nivolumab Sponsor: Indications.*; 2014. https://www.accessdata.fda.gov/drugsatfda_docs/nda/2014/125554Orig1s000Approv.pdf
7. Merck. Ten-Year Data for Merck's KEYTRUDA® (pembrolizumab) Demonstrates Sustained Overall Survival Benefit Versus Ipilimumab in Advanced Melanoma - Merck.com. Merck.com. Published October 13, 2024. https://www.merck.com/news/ten-year-data-for-mercks-keytruda-pembrolizumab-demonstrates-sustained-overall-survival-benefit-versus-ipilimumab-in-advanced-melanoma/
8. Drug Approval Package: Brand Name (Generic Name) NDA #. www.accessdata.fda.gov.

https://www.accessdata.fda.gov/drugsatfda_docs/nda/2011/125377Orig1s000TOC.cfm

9. Cancer Research Institute. She's the Answer to Cancer...and So Are You. YouTube. Published May 6, 2016. Accessed December 3, 2024. https://www.youtube.com/watch?v=0Yw0GaKTkxE

10. A Complete Response: Sharon's Story. MSK Giving. Published May 13, 2021. https://giving.mskcc.org/complete-response-sharons-story

11. Choi J, Lee SY. Clinical Characteristics and Treatment of Immune-Related Adverse Events of Immune Checkpoint Inhibitors. *Immune Network.* 2020;20(1). doi:https://doi.org/10.4110/in.2020.20.e9

12. Fecher LA, Agarwala SS, Hodi FS, Weber JS. Ipilimumab and Its Toxicities: A Multidisciplinary Approach. *The Oncologist.* 2013;18(6):733-743. doi:https://doi.org/10.1634/theoncologist.2012-0483

13. Lechner MG, Zhou Z, Hoang AT, et al. Clonally expanded, thyrotoxic effector CD8 + T cells driven by IL-21 contribute to checkpoint inhibitor thyroiditis. *Science translational medicine.* 2023;15(696). doi:https://doi.org/10.1126/scitranslmed.adg0675

14. Kotwal A, Haddox C, Block M, Kudva YC. Immune checkpoint inhibitors: an emerging cause of insulin-dependent diabetes. *BMJ Open Diabetes Research & Care.* 2019;7(1):e000591. doi:https://doi.org/10.1136/bmjdrc-2018-000591

15. Blum SM, Zlotoff DA, Smith NP, et al. Immune responses in checkpoint myocarditis across heart, blood and tumour. *Nature*. Published online November 6, 2024:1-9. doi:https://doi.org/10.1038/s41586-024-08105-5

16. Johnson DB, Sullivan RJ, Ott PA, et al. Ipilimumab Therapy in Patients With Advanced Melanoma and Preexisting Autoimmune Disorders. *JAMA Oncology*. 2016;2(2):234. doi:https://doi.org/10.1001/jamaoncol.2015.4368

17. Blum SM, Zlotoff DA, Smith NP, et al. Immune responses in checkpoint myocarditis across heart, blood and tumour. *Nature*. Published online November 6, 2024:1-9. doi:https://doi.org/10.1038/s41586-024-08105-5

18. Dai WF, Beca JM, Croxford R, et al. Real-world comparative effectiveness of second-line ipilimumab for metastatic melanoma: a population-based cohort study in Ontario, Canada. *BMC Cancer*. 2020;20(1). doi:https://doi.org/10.1186/s12885-020-06798-1

19. Dalle S, Mortier L, Corrie P, et al. Long-term real-world experience with ipilimumab and non-ipilimumab therapies in advanced melanoma: the IMAGE study. *BMC Cancer*. 2021;21(1). doi:https://doi.org/10.1186/s12885-021-08032-y

20. Long GV, Carlino MS, McNeil C, et al. Pembrolizumab versus ipilimumab for advanced melanoma: 10-year follow-up of the phase III KEYNOTE-006 study. *Annals of Oncology*. Published online September 15, 2024. doi:https://doi.org/10.1016/j.annonc.2024.08.2330

21. Allison J. Melanoma survivor Sharon Belvin meets Dr. Jim Allison for the first time. Cancer History Project. Published 2023. https://cancerhistoryproject.com/article/melanoma-survivor-sharon-belvin-meets-dr-jim-allison-for-the-first-time/

22. Garbe C, Eigentler TK, Keilholz U, Hauschild A, Kirkwood JM. Systematic Review of Medical Treatment in Melanoma: Current Status and Future Prospects. *The Oncologist.* 2011;16(1):5-24. doi:https://doi.org/10.1634/theoncologist.2010-0190

23. *HIGHLIGHTS of PRESCRIBING INFORMATION.*; 2022. https://www.accessdata.fda.gov/drugsatfda_docs/label/2022/761289lbl.pdf

24. Raedler LA. Keytruda (Pembrolizumab): First PD-1 Inhibitor Approved for Previously Treated Unresectable or Metastatic Melanoma. *American Health & Drug Benefits.* 2015;8(Spec Feature):96. https://pmc.ncbi.nlm.nih.gov/articles/PMC4665064/

25. Bristol-Myers Squibb Receives Accelerated Approval of Opdivo (nivolumab) from the U.S. Food and Drug Administration. Bms.com. Published 2020. Accessed December 3, 2024. https://news.bms.com/news/details/2014/Bristol-Myers-Squibb-Receives-Accelerated-Approval-of-Opdivo-nivolumab-from-the-US-Food-and-Drug-Administration/default.aspx

26. *CENTER for DRUG EVALUATION and RESEARCH Approval Package For.* https://www.accessdata.fda.gov/drugsatfda_docs/nda/2014/125514Orig1s000Approv.pdf

27. Myers B. *CENTER for DRUG EVALUATION and RESEARCH Approval Package For: APPLICATION NUMBER: 125554Orig1s000 Trade Name: Opdivo Generic Name: Nivolumab Sponsor: Indications.*; 2014. https://www.accessdata.fda.gov/drugsatfda_docs/nda/2014/125554Orig1s000Approv.pdf

28. Martins F, Sofiya L, Sykiotis GP, et al. Adverse effects of immune-checkpoint inhibitors: epidemiology, management and surveillance. *Nature Reviews Clinical Oncology.* 2019;16(9):563-580. doi:https://doi.org/10.1038/s41571-019-0218-0

29. Morelli T, Fujita K, Redelman-Sidi G, Elkington PT. Infections due to dysregulated immunity: an emerging complication of cancer immunotherapy. *Thorax.* 2022;77(3):304-311. doi:https://doi.org/10.1136/thoraxjnl-2021-217260

30. Ogishi M, Kitaoka K, Good-Jacobson KL, et al. Impaired development of memory B cells and antibody responses in humans and mice deficient in PD-1 signaling. *Immunity.* Published online November 2024. doi:https://doi.org/10.1016/j.immuni.2024.10.014

31. Wolchok JD, Chiarion-Sileni V, Gonzalez R, et al. Long-Term Outcomes With Nivolumab Plus Ipilimumab or Nivolumab Alone Versus Ipilimumab in Patients With

Advanced Melanoma. *Journal of Clinical Oncology*. 2021;40(2). doi:https://doi.org/10.1200/jco.21.02229

32. Not van, van, Jalving H, et al. Long-Term Survival in Patients With Advanced Melanoma. *JAMA Network Open*. 2024;7(8):e2426641-e2426641. doi:https://doi.org/10.1001/jamanetworkopen.2024.26641

33. Rivera MP, Mehta AC, Wahidi MM. Establishing the Diagnosis of Lung Cancer. *Chest*. 2013;143(5):e142Se165S. doi:https://doi.org/10.1378/chest.12-2353

34. Anita: Lung Cancer Survivor. Yale Medicine. https://www.yalemedicine.org/survivor-stories/anita-thoracic-cancer-survivor

35. Legacy. Anita Adler Obituary (1938 - 2020) - New London, CT - The Day. Legacy.com. Published June 2, 2020. Accessed December 3, 2024. https://www.legacy.com/us/obituaries/theday/name/anita-adler-obituary?id=8589342

36. J. Davies, DNP, MSN, RN, APRN, CNS-BC, ACNP-BC, AOCNP M. PD-1/PD-L1 Inhibitors for Non–Small Cell Lung Cancer: Incorporating Care Step Pathways for Effective Side-Effect Management. *Journal of the Advanced Practitioner in Oncology*. 2019;10(2). doi:https://doi.org/10.6004/jadpro.2019.10.2.11

37. Reck M, Rodríguez-Abreu D, Robinson AG, et al. Five-Year Outcomes With Pembrolizumab Versus Chemotherapy for Metastatic Non–Small-Cell Lung Cancer With PD-L1 Tumor Proportion Score ≥ 50%.

Journal of Clinical Oncology. 2021;39(21):JCO.21.00174. doi:https://doi.org/10.1200/jco.21.00174

38. Research C for DE and. Atezolizumab (TECENTRIQ). *FDA*. Published online November 3, 2018. https://www.fda.gov/drugs/resources-information-approved-drugs/atezolizumab-tecentriq

39. Research C for DE and. Durvalumab (Imfinzi). *FDA*. Published online February 9, 2019. https://www.fda.gov/drugs/resources-information-approved-drugs/durvalumab-imfinzi

40. Research C for DE and. Avelumab (BAVENCIO). *FDA*. Published online February 9, 2019. https://www.fda.gov/drugs/resources-information-approved-drugs/avelumab-bavencio

41. Pillai RN, Behera M, Owonikoko TK, et al. Comparison of the toxicity profile of PD-1 versus PD-L1 inhibitors in non-small cell lung cancer: A systematic analysis of the literature. *Cancer*. 2017;124(2):271-277. doi:https://doi.org/10.1002/cncr.31043

42. De Sousa Linhares A, Battin C, Jutz S, et al. Therapeutic PD-L1 antibodies are more effective than PD-1 antibodies in blocking PD-1/PD-L1 signaling. *Scientific Reports*. 2019;9(1). doi:https://doi.org/10.1038/s41598-019-47910-1

43. Andrews LP, Cillo AR, Karapetyan L, Kirkwood JM, Workman CJ, Vignali DAA. Molecular Pathways and Mechanisms of LAG3 in Cancer Therapy. *Clinical Cancer Research*. 2022;28(23):5030-5039. doi:https://doi.org/10.1158/1078-0432.ccr-21-2390

44. Sauer N, Wojciech Szlasa, Jonderko L, et al. LAG-3 as a Potent Target for Novel Anticancer Therapies of a Wide Range of Tumors. *Scientific Discoveries Supporting Theories in Science: From Thinking to Practice.* 2022;23(17):9958-9958. doi:https://doi.org/10.3390/ijms23179958

45. Huo JL, Wang YT, Fu WJ, Lu N, Liu ZS. The promising immune checkpoint LAG-3 in cancer immunotherapy: from basic research to clinical application. *Frontiers in Immunology*. 2022;13. doi:https://doi.org/10.3389/fimmu.2022.956090

46. Orcione R. Melanoma Clinical Trial Success Story: From Patient Volunteer to No Evidence of Disease. Melanoma Research Alliance. Published 2022. Accessed December 3, 2024. https://www.curemelanoma.org/blog/article/melanoma-clinical-trial-success-story-from-patient-volunteer-to-no-evidence-of-disease

47. Inman BA, Longo TA, Ramalingam S, Harrison MR. Atezolizumab: A PD-L1-Blocking Antibody for Bladder Cancer. *Clinical cancer research : an official journal of the American Association for Cancer Research.* 2017;23(8):1886-1890. doi:https://doi.org/10.1158/1078-0432.CCR-16-1417

48. D'Angelo SP, Russell J, Lebbé C, et al. Efficacy and Safety of First-line Avelumab Treatment in Patients With Stage IV Metastatic Merkel Cell Carcinoma. *JAMA Oncology*.

2018;4(9):e180077. doi:https://doi.org/10.1001/jamaoncol.2018.0077

49. Bhatia S, Nghiem P, Veeranki SP, et al. Real-world clinical outcomes with avelumab in patients with Merkel cell carcinoma treated in the USA: a multicenter chart review study. *Journal for ImmunoTherapy of Cancer.* 2022;10(8):e004904. doi:https://doi.org/10.1136/jitc-2022-004904

50. D'Angelo SP, Bhatia S, Brohl AS, et al. Avelumab in patients with previously treated metastatic Merkel cell carcinoma: long-term data and biomarker analyses from the single-arm phase 2 JAVELIN Merkel 200 trial. *Journal for ImmunoTherapy of Cancer.* 2020;8(1):e000674. doi:https://doi.org/10.1136/jitc-2020-000674

Chapter 6

1. Amjad MT, Kasi A, Chidharla A. Cancer Chemotherapy. PubMed. Published February 27, 2023. https://www.ncbi.nlm.nih.gov/books/NBK564367/

2. Institute of Cancer Reasearh London. Science Talk - "Immunotherapy is keeping me alive" - John's story - The Institute of Cancer Research, London. Icr.ac.uk. Published 2023. https://www.icr.ac.uk/blogs/science-talk/page-details/immunotherapy-is-keeping-me-alive---john-s-story

3. Blank CU, Blank CU, Blank CU, et al. Neoadjuvant Nivolumab and Ipilimumab in Resectable Stage III Melanoma. *New England journal of medicine/The New*

England journal of medicine. Published online June 2, 2024. doi:https://doi.org/10.1056/nejmoa2402604

4. Wolchok JD, Chiarion-Sileni V, Gonzalez R, et al. Overall Survival with Combined Nivolumab and Ipilimumab in Advanced Melanoma. *New England Journal of Medicine.* 2017;377(14):1345-1356. doi:https://doi.org/10.1056/nejmoa1709684
5. Redirecting. Elsevier.com. Published 2024. Accessed November 21, 2024. https://linkinghub.elsevier.com/retrieve/pii/S0305737216000165
6. Godwin JW, Jaggi S, Imali Sirisena, et al. Nivolumab-induced autoimmune diabetes mellitus presenting as diabetic ketoacidosis in a patient with metastatic lung cancer. 2017;5(1). doi:https://doi.org/10.1186/s40425-017-0245-2
7. Wu X, Sun Y, Yang H, et al. Cadonilimab plus platinum-based chemotherapy with or without bevacizumab as first-line treatment for persistent, recurrent, or metastatic cervical cancer (COMPASSION-16): a randomised, double-blind, placebo-controlled phase 3 trial in China. *The Lancet.* 2024;404(10463):1668-1676. doi:https://doi.org/10.1016/s0140-6736(24)02135-4
8. Wolters Kluwer. Ovid.com. Published 2024. Accessed November 21, 2024. https://oce.ovid.com/article/00005083-202206011-04411?relatedarticle=y
9. Angeles. Combination approach shows promise for treating rare, aggressive cancers. Medicalxpress.com. Published

November 12, 2024. Accessed November 21, 2024. https://medicalxpress.com/news/2024-11-combination-approach-rare-aggressive-cancers.html

10. Gu Y, Ly A, Rodriguez S, et al. PD-1 blockade plus cisplatin-based chemotherapy in patients with small cell/neuroendocrine bladder and prostate cancers. *Cell Reports Medicine*. 2024;5(11):101824. doi:https://doi.org/10.1016/j.xcrm.2024.101824

11. Gennigens C. Hope emerging in the locally advanced cervical cancer landscape. *The Lancet*. Published online September 1, 2024. doi:https://doi.org/10.1016/s0140-6736(24)01918-4

12. Jin Y, Wei J, Weng Y, et al. Adjuvant Therapy With PD1/PDL1 Inhibitors for Human Cancers: A Systematic Review and Meta-Analysis. *Frontiers in Oncology*. 2022;12. doi:https://doi.org/10.3389/fonc.2022.732814

13. García-González J, Ruiz-Bañobre J, Afonso-Afonso FJ, et al. PD-(L)1 Inhibitors in Combination with Chemotherapy as First-Line Treatment for Non-Small-Cell Lung Cancer: A Pairwise Meta-Analysis. *Journal of Clinical Medicine*. 2020;9(7):2093. doi:https://doi.org/10.3390/jcm9072093

14. Shao T, Zhao M, Liang L, Tang W. A systematic review and network meta-analysis of first-line immune checkpoint inhibitor combination therapies in patients with advanced non-squamous non-small cell lung cancer. *Elsevier*. 2022;13(2). doi:https://doi.org/10.3389/fimmu.2022.948597

15. Rizvi NA, Ademuyiwa FO, Z. Alexander Cao, et al. Society for Immunotherapy of Cancer (SITC) consensus

definitions for resistance to combinations of immune checkpoint inhibitors with chemotherapy. *Journal for ImmunoTherapy of Cancer.* 2023;11(3):e005920-e005920. doi:https://doi.org/10.1136/jitc-2022-005920

16. Wu L, Zhang Z, Bai M, Yan Y, Yu J, Xu Y. Radiation combined with immune checkpoint inhibitors for unresectable locally advanced non-small cell lung cancer: synergistic mechanisms, current state, challenges, and orientations. *Cell Communication and Signaling.* 2023;21(1). doi:https://doi.org/10.1186/s12964-023-01139-8
17. Yan Y, Kumar AB, Finnes H, et al. Combining Immune Checkpoint Inhibitors With Conventional Cancer Therapy. *Frontiers in Immunology.* 2018;9. doi:https://doi.org/10.3389/fimmu.2018.01739
18. Wang F, Yang S, Palmer N, et al. Real-world data analyses unveiled the immune-related adverse effects of immune checkpoint inhibitors across cancer types. *npj Precision Oncology.* 2021;5(1):1-11. doi:https://doi.org/10.1038/s41698-021-00223-x
19. Greeshma Rajeev-Kumar, Pitroda SP. Synergizing radiotherapy and immunotherapy: Current challenges and strategies for optimization. *Neoplasia.* 2023;36:100867-100867. doi:https://doi.org/10.1016/j.neo.2022.100867
20. Meng L, Xu J, Ye Y, Wang Y, Luo S, Gong X. The Combination of Radiotherapy With Immunotherapy and Potential Predictive Biomarkers for Treatment of Non-Small Cell Lung Cancer Patients. *Frontiers in*

Immunology. 2021;12. doi:https://doi.org/10.3389/fimmu.2021.723609

21. Shaverdian N, Lisberg AE, Bornazyan K, et al. Previous radiotherapy and the clinical activity and toxicity of pembrolizumab in the treatment of non-small-cell lung cancer: a secondary analysis of the KEYNOTE-001 phase 1 trial. *The Lancet Oncology*. 2017;18(7):895-903. doi:https://doi.org/10.1016/S1470-2045(17)30380-7
22. Fukushima H, Toshiki Kijima, Fukuda S, et al. Impact of radiotherapy to the primary tumor on the efficacy of pembrolizumab for patients with advanced urothelial cancer: A preliminary study. *Cancer Medicine*. 2020;9(22):8355-8363. doi:https://doi.org/10.1002/cam4.3445
23. Wu L, Zhang Z, Bai M, Yan Y, Yu J, Xu Y. Radiation combined with immune checkpoint inhibitors for unresectable locally advanced non-small cell lung cancer: synergistic mechanisms, current state, challenges, and orientations. *Cell Communication and Signaling*. 2023;21(1). doi:https://doi.org/10.1186/s12964-023-01139-8
24. Li B, Jin J, Guo D, Tao Z, Hu X. Immune Checkpoint Inhibitors Combined with Targeted Therapy: The Recent Advances and Future Potentials. *Cancers*. 2023;15(10):2858. doi:https://doi.org/10.3390/cancers15102858
25. Li B, Jin J, Guo D, Tao Z, Hu X. Immune Checkpoint Inhibitors Combined with Targeted Therapy: The Recent Advances and Future Potentials. *Cancers*.

2023;15(10):2858. doi:https://doi.org/10.3390/cancers15102858

26. Atkins MB, Plimack ER, Puzanov I, et al. Axitinib in combination with pembrolizumab in patients with advanced renal cell cancer: a non-randomised, open-label, dose-finding, and dose-expansion phase 1b trial. *The Lancet Oncology*. 2018;19(3):405-415. doi:https://doi.org/10.1016/s1470-2045(18)30081-0

27. Walsh RJ, Sundar R, Lim JSJ. Immune checkpoint inhibitor combinations—current and emerging strategies. *British Journal of Cancer*. Published online February 6, 2023. doi:https://doi.org/10.1038/s41416-023-02181-6

28. Tawbi HA, Hodi FS, Lipson EJ, et al. Nivolumab (NIVO) plus relatlimab (RELA) vs NIVO in previously untreated metastatic or unresectable melanoma (RELATIVITY-047): Overall survival (OS) and melanoma-specific survival (MSS) outcomes at 3 years. *Journal of Clinical Oncology*. 2024;42(16_suppl):9524-9524. doi:https://doi.org/10.1200/jco.2024.42.16_suppl.9524

29. *HIGHLIGHTS of PRESCRIBING INFORMATION*. https://www.accessdata.fda.gov/drugsatfda_docs/label/2022/761289lbl.pdf

30. Curran MA, Montalvo W, Yagita H, Allison JP. PD-1 and CTLA-4 combination blockade expands infiltrating T cells and reduces regulatory T and myeloid cells within B16 melanoma tumors. *Proceedings of the National Academy of Sciences*. 2010;107(9):4275-4280. doi:https://doi.org/10.1073/pnas.0915174107

31. Wolchok JD, Chiarion-Sileni V, Gonzalez R, et al. Long-Term Outcomes With Nivolumab Plus Ipilimumab or Nivolumab Alone Versus Ipilimumab in Patients With Advanced Melanoma. *Journal of Clinical Oncology.* 2021;40(2). doi:https://doi.org/10.1200/jco.21.02229

32. Nishio M, Ohe Y, Ikeda S, et al. First-line nivolumab plus ipilimumab in metastatic non-small cell lung cancer: 5-year outcomes in Japanese patients from CheckMate 227 Part 1. *International Journal of Clinical Oncology.* 2023;28(10):1354-1368. doi:https://doi.org/10.1007/s10147-023-02390-2

33. Nishio M, Ohe Y, Ikeda S, et al. First-line nivolumab plus ipilimumab in metastatic non-small cell lung cancer: 5-year outcomes in Japanese patients from CheckMate 227 Part 1. *International Journal of Clinical Oncology.* 2023;28(10):1354-1368. doi:https://doi.org/10.1007/s10147-023-02390-2

34. Nakamura Y, Namikawa K, Yoshikawa S, et al. Anti-PD-1 antibody monotherapy versus anti-PD-1 plus anti-CTLA-4 combination therapy as first-line immunotherapy in unresectable or metastatic mucosal melanoma: a retrospective, multicenter study of 329 Japanese cases (JMAC study). *ESMO Open.* 2021;6(6):100325. doi:https://doi.org/10.1016/j.esmoop.2021.100325

35. Klein-Brill A, Amar-Farkash S, Rosenberg-Katz K, Brenner R, Becker JC, Aran D. Comparative efficacy of combined CTLA-4 and PD-1 blockade vs. PD-1 monotherapy in metastatic melanoma: a real-world study. *BJC Reports.*

2024;2(1):1-7. doi:https://doi.org/10.1038/s44276-024-00041-1

36. Martini DJ, Lalani AKA, Bosse D, et al. Response to single agent PD-1 inhibitor after progression on previous PD-1/PD-L1 inhibitors: a case series . Bmj.com. Published 2017. Accessed December 6, 2024. https://jitc.bmj.com/content/5/1/66

37. 330.

38. Harris NL, Ronchese F. The role of B7 costimulation in T-cell immunity. *Immunology and Cell Biology*. 1999;77(4):304-311. doi:https://doi.org/10.1046/j.1440-1711.1999.00835.x

39. Voss MH, Azad AA, Hansen AR, et al. A Randomized Phase II Study of MEDI0680 in Combination with Durvalumab versus Nivolumab Monotherapy in Patients with Advanced or Metastatic Clear-cell Renal Cell Carcinoma. *Clinical Cancer Research*. 2022;28(14):3032-3041. doi:https://doi.org/10.1158/1078-0432.ccr-21-4115

40. Ankit Mangla, Lee C, Mirsky MM, et al. Neoadjuvant Dual Checkpoint Inhibitors vs Anti-PD1 Therapy in High-Risk Resectable Melanoma. *JAMA Oncology*. 2024;10(5):612-612. doi:https://doi.org/10.1001/jamaoncol.2023.7333

41. Kong X, Lu P, Liu C, et al. A combination of PD-1/PD-L1 inhibitors: The prospect of overcoming the weakness of tumor immunotherapy (Review). *Molecular Medicine Reports*. 2021;23(5). doi:https://doi.org/10.3892/mmr.2021.12001

42. Yufan Lv, Luo X, Xie Z, et al. Prospects and challenges of CAR-T cell therapy combined with ICIs. *Frontiers in oncology*. 2024;14. doi:https://doi.org/10.3389/fonc.2024.1368732

43. Zhou D, Zhu X, Xiao Y. CAR-T cell combination therapies in hematologic malignancies. *Experimental Hematology and Oncology*. 2024;13(1). doi:https://doi.org/10.1186/s40164-024-00536-0

44. A Chong E, Svoboda J, Dwivedy Nasta S, et al. Sequential Anti-CD19 Directed Chimeric Antigen Receptor Modified T-Cell Therapy (CART19) and PD-1 Blockade with Pembrolizumab in Patients with Relapsed or Refractory B-Cell Non-Hodgkin Lymphomas. *Blood*. 2018;132(supplement 1).

Chapter 7

1. Harms PW, Harms KL, Moore PS, et al. The biology and treatment of Merkel cell carcinoma: current understanding and research priorities. *Nature Reviews Clinical Oncology*. 2018;15(12):763-776. doi:https://doi.org/10.1038/s41571-018-0103-2

2. Merkel Cell Carcinoma (MCC). Yale Medicine. https://www.yalemedicine.org/conditions/merkel-cell-carcinoma-mcc

3. Survival Rates for Merkel Cell Carcinoma. www.cancer.org. https://www.cancer.org/cancer/types/merkel-cell-skin-cancer/detection-diagnosis-staging/survival-rates.html

4. Pancreatic Cancer Facts. Hirshberg Foundation for Pancreatic Cancer Research. https://pancreatic.org/pancreatic-cancer/pancreatic-cancer-facts/

5. Jančík S, Drábek J, Radzioch D, Hajdúch M. Clinical Relevance of KRAS in Human Cancers. *Journal of Biomedicine and Biotechnology*. 2010;2010:1-13. doi:https://doi.org/10.1155/2010/150960

6. Mekapogu A, Srinivasa Pothula, Romano Pirola, Wilson J, Apte M. Pancreatic Stellate Cells in Health and Disease. Published online November 19, 2020. doi:https://doi.org/10.3998/panc.2020.08

7. Murphy S. Identifying inherited gene mutations in pancreatic cancer can lead to targeted therapies, better survival - Mayo Clinic News Network. Mayo Clinic News Network. Published November 24, 2022. Accessed November 21, 2024. https://newsnetwork.mayoclinic.org/discussion/science-saturday-identifying-inherited-gene-mutations-in-pancreatic-cancer-can-lead-to-targeted-therapies-better-survival/

8. Jain A, Bhardwaj V. Therapeutic resistance in pancreatic ductal adenocarcinoma: Current challenges and future opportunities. *World Journal of Gastroenterology*. 2021;27(39):6527-6550. doi:https://doi.org/10.3748/wjg.v27.i39.6527

9. Deniz Can Guven, Gozde Kavgaci, Enes Erul, et al. The Efficacy of Immune Checkpoint Inhibitors in

Microsatellite Stable Colorectal Cancer: A Systematic Review. *The oncologist.* Published online February 3, 2024. doi:https://doi.org/10.1093/oncolo/oyae013

10. In a First, Immune Checkpoint Inhibitors Show Effectiveness in Metastatic Colorectal Cancer - Dana-Farber. Dana-farber.org. Published July 24, 2024. Accessed November 21, 2024. https://physicianresources.dana-farber.org/news/in-a-first-immune-checkpoint-inhibitors-show-effectiveness-in-metastatic-colorectal-cancer
11. Yu J, Wang X, Teng F, Kong L. PD-L1 expression in human cancers and its association with clinical outcomes. *OncoTargets and Therapy.* 2016;Volume 9:5023-5039. doi:https://doi.org/10.2147/ott.s105862
12. Tang Q, Chen Y, Li X, et al. The role of PD-1/PD-L1 and application of immune-checkpoint inhibitors in human cancers. *Frontiers in Immunology.* 2022;13:964442. doi:https://doi.org/10.3389/fimmu.2022.964442
13. Yoon SB, Woo SM, Chun JW, et al. The predictive value of PD-L1 expression in response to anti-PD-1/PD-L1 therapy for biliary tract cancer: a systematic review and meta-analysis. *Frontiers in Immunology.* 2024;15. doi:https://doi.org/10.3389/fimmu.2024.1321813
14. Patel SP, Kurzrock R. PD-L1 Expression as a Predictive Biomarker in Cancer Immunotherapy. *Molecular Cancer Therapeutics.* 2015;14(4):847-856. doi:https://doi.org/10.1158/1535-7163.mct-14-0983
15. Rubio-Viqueira B, Tarruella MM, Lázaro M, et al. PD-L1 testing and clinical management of newly diagnosed

metastatic non-small cell lung cancer in Spain: MOREL study. *Lung Cancer Management.* 2021;10(4). doi:https://doi.org/10.2217/lmt-2021-0008

16. Flaherty C. PD-L1 Expression Remains Primary Guide for NSCLC Treatment Selection in the Absence of Targetable Mutations. OncLive. Published August 5, 2024. Accessed November 21, 2024. https://www.onclive.com/view/pd-l1-expression-remains-primary-guide-for-nsclc-treatment-selection-in-the-absence-of-targetable-mutations
17. Tumor Mutational Burden | TMB NGS testing. Illumina.com. Published 2020. Accessed November 21, 2024. https://www.illumina.com/areas-of-interest/cancer/ngs-in-oncology/biomarkers/tumor-mutational-burden.html
18. Budczies J, Kazdal D, Menzel M, et al. Tumour mutational burden: clinical utility, challenges and emerging improvements. *Nature Reviews Clinical Oncology.* 2024;21(10):725-742. doi:https://doi.org/10.1038/s41571-024-00932-9
19. Lu C, Liu Y, Ali NM, Zhang B, Cui X. The role of innate immune cells in the tumor microenvironment and research progress in anti-tumor therapy. *Frontiers in Immunology.* 2023;13. doi:https://doi.org/10.3389/fimmu.2022.1039260
20. NCI Dictionary of Cancer Terms. National Cancer Institute. Published 2019. https://www.cancer.gov/publications/dictionaries/cancer-terms/def/tumor-microenvironment

21. Anderson NM, Simon MC. The Tumor Microenvironment. *Current Biology*. 2020;30(16):R921-R925. doi:https://doi.org/10.1016/j.cub.2020.06.081

22. Schmidt A, Oberle N, Krammer PH. Molecular Mechanisms of Treg-Mediated T Cell Suppression. *Frontiers in Immunology*. 2012;3. doi:https://doi.org/10.3389/fimmu.2012.00051

23. LV B, Wang Y, Ma D, et al. Immunotherapy: Reshape the Tumor Immune Microenvironment. *Frontiers in Immunology*. 2022;13. doi:https://doi.org/10.3389/fimmu.2022.844142

24. Gut Bacteria Affect Immunotherapy Response. National Cancer Institute. Published February 5, 2018. https://www.cancer.gov/news-events/cancer-currents-blog/2018/gut-bacteria-checkpoint-inhibitors

25. Lee KA, Thomas AM, Bolte LA, et al. Cross-cohort gut microbiome associations with immune checkpoint inhibitor response in advanced melanoma. *Nature Medicine*. Published online February 28, 2022:1-10. doi:https://doi.org/10.1038/s41591-022-01695-5

26. Gopalakrishnan V, Spencer CN, Nezi L, et al. Gut microbiome modulates response to anti–PD-1 immunotherapy in melanoma patients. *Science*. 2017;359(6371):97-103. doi:https://doi.org/10.1126/science.aan4236

27. Routy B, Le Chatelier E, Derosa L, et al. Gut microbiome influences efficacy of PD-1-based immunotherapy against epithelial tumors. *Science (New York, NY)*.

2018;359(6371):91-97. doi:https://doi.org/10.1126/science.aan3706

28. Matson V, Fessler J, Bao R, et al. The commensal microbiome is associated with anti–PD-1 efficacy in metastatic melanoma patients. *Science*. 2018;359(6371):104-108. doi:https://doi.org/10.1126/science.aao3290

29. Zhang M, Liu J, Xia Q. Role of gut microbiome in cancer immunotherapy: from predictive biomarker to therapeutic target. *Experimental Hematology & Oncology*. 2023;12(1). doi:https://doi.org/10.1186/s40164-023-00442-x

30. Kim CH. Complex regulatory effects of gut microbial short-chain fatty acids on immune tolerance and autoimmunity. *Cellular & Molecular Immunology*. 2023;20(4):341-350. doi:https://doi.org/10.1038/s41423-023-00987-1

31. Lee KA, Thomas AM, Bolte LA, et al. Cross-cohort gut microbiome associations with immune checkpoint inhibitor response in advanced melanoma. *Nature Medicine*. Published online February 28, 2022:1-10. doi:https://doi.org/10.1038/s41591-022-01695-5

32. Turning cold tumors hot: Drug delivery system makes immunotherapy more effective. Uchicago.edu. Published April 14, 2020. Accessed November 21, 2024. https://pme.uchicago.edu/news/turning-cold-tumors-hot-drug-delivery-system-makes-immunotherapy-more-effective

33. Targeted Therapy Drug List by Cancer Type - NCI. www.cancer.gov. Published October 3, 2022.

https://www.cancer.gov/about-cancer/treatment/types/targeted-therapies/approved-drug-list

34. Turning cold tumors hot: Drug delivery system makes immunotherapy more effective. Uchicago.edu. Published April 14, 2020. Accessed November 21, 2024. https://pme.uchicago.edu/news/turning-cold-tumors-hot-drug-delivery-system-makes-immunotherapy-more-effective
35. Ouyang P, Wang L, Wu J, et al. Overcoming cold tumors: a combination strategy of immune checkpoint inhibitors. *Frontiers in immunology*. 2024;15. doi:https://doi.org/10.3389/fimmu.2024.1344272
36. Liu YT, Sun ZJ. Turning cold tumors into hot tumors by improving T-cell infiltration. *Theranostics*. 2021;11(11):5365-5386. doi:https://doi.org/10.7150/thno.58390
37. Wu YY, Sun TK, Chen MS, Munir M, Liu HJ. Oncolytic viruses-modulated immunogenic cell death, apoptosis and autophagy linking to virotherapy and cancer immune response. *Frontiers in Cellular and Infection Microbiology*. 2023;13. doi:https://doi.org/10.3389/fcimb.2023.1142172
38. National Cancer Institute. Using Oncolytic Viruses to Treat Cancer. National Cancer Institute. Published February 9, 2018. https://www.cancer.gov/news-events/cancer-currents-blog/2018/oncolytic-viruses-to-treat-cancer
39. Chehelgerdi M, Matin Chehelgerdi, Omer Qutaiba Al-lela, et al. Progressing nanotechnology to improve targeted

cancer treatment: overcoming hurdles in its clinical implementation. *Molecular Cancer.* 2023;22(1). doi:https://doi.org/10.1186/s12943-023-01865-0

Chapter 8

1. Roche. Roche | What is a liquid biopsy? www.roche.com. https://www.roche.com/stories/liquid-biopsy-in-oncology
2. Liquid biopsy: A new tool for identifying and monitoring cancer. www.uchicagomedicine.org. https://www.uchicagomedicine.org/forefront/cancer-articles/liquid-biopsies
3. Kwong GA, Ghosh S, Gamboa L, Patriotis C, Srivastava S, Bhatia SN. Synthetic biomarkers: a twenty-first century path to early cancer detection. *Nature Reviews Cancer.* 2021;21(10):655-668. doi:https://doi.org/10.1038/s41568-021-00389-3
4. PhD SL. The Expanding Potential of Liquid Biopsy to Detect and Monitor Cancer. American Association for Cancer Research (AACR). Published August 31, 2023. https://www.aacr.org/blog/2023/08/31/the-expanding-potential-of-liquid-biopsy-to-detect-and-monitor-cancer/
5. UChicago scientists decode key mutation in many cancers. University of Chicago News. Published October 2, 2024. https://news.uchicago.edu/story/uchicago-scientists-decode-key-mutation-many-cancers
6. Locke WJ, Guanzon D, Ma C, et al. DNA Methylation Cancer Biomarkers: Translation to the Clinic. *Frontiers in*

Genetics. 2019;10. doi:https://doi.org/10.3389/fgene.2019.01150

7. Kwon H, Sun Hye Shin, Hyun Ho Kim, et al. Advances in methylation analysis of liquid biopsy in early cancer detection of colorectal and lung cancer. *Scientific Reports*. 2023;13(1). doi:https://doi.org/10.1038/s41598-023-40611-w

8. Cristiano S, Leal A, Phallen J, et al. Genome-wide cell-free DNA fragmentation in patients with cancer. *Nature*. 2019;570(7761):385-389. doi:https://doi.org/10.1038/s41586-019-1272-6

9. Connal S, Cameron JM, Sala A, et al. Liquid biopsies: the future of cancer early detection. *Journal of Translational Medicine*. 2023;21(1). doi:https://doi.org/10.1186/s12967-023-03960-8

10. Hayashi H, Chamoto K, Hatae R, et al. Soluble immune checkpoint factors reflect exhaustion of antitumor immunity and response to PD-1 blockade. *The Journal of Clinical Investigation*. 2024;134(7). doi:https://doi.org/10.1172/JCI168318

11. Beyond Liquid Biopsies: How the Synthetic Biopsy Leads the Next Generation of Early Cancer Detection. www.earli.com. https://www.earli.com/post/beyond-liquid-biopsies-how-the-synthetic-biopsy-leads-the-next-generation-of-early-cancer-detection

12. Kwong GA, Ghosh S, Gamboa L, Patriotis C, Srivastava S, Bhatia SN. Synthetic biomarkers: a twenty-first century path to early cancer detection. *Nature Reviews Cancer*.

2021;21(10):655-668. doi:https://doi.org/10.1038/s41568-021-00389-3

13. AI Outperformed Standard Risk Model for Predicting Breast Cancer. www.rsna.org. Published June 6, 2023. https://www.rsna.org/news/2023/june/ai-for-predicting-breast-cancer

14. Santeramo R, Damiani C, Wei J, Montana G, Brentnall AR. Are better AI algorithms for breast cancer detection also better at predicting risk? A paired case–control study. *Breast Cancer Research*. 2024;26(1). doi:https://doi.org/10.1186/s13058-024-01775-z

15. MIT. SYBIL – MIT Jameel Clinic. Mit.edu. Published 2024. Accessed November 21, 2024. https://jclinic.mit.edu/sybil/

16. MIT researchers develop an AI model that can detect future lung cancer risk | LCFA. LCFA. Published December 18, 2023. Accessed November 21, 2024. https://lcfamerica.org/research-news/mit-researchers-develop-an-ai-model-that-can-detect-future-lung-cancer-risk/

17. Glasgow G. CU Cancer Center Helps Lead National Trial to Evaluate Multicancer Blood Tests. Cuanschutz.edu. Published April 18, 2024. https://news.cuanschutz.edu/cancer-center/national-trial-to-evaluate-multicancer-blood-tests

18. Questions and Answers about MCD Tests. prevention.cancer.gov. https://prevention.cancer.gov/major-

programs/multi-cancer-detection-mcd-research/questions-and-answers-about-mcd-tests

19. Zahavi DJ, Weiner LM. Targeting Multiple Receptors to Increase Checkpoint Blockade Efficacy. *International Journal of Molecular Sciences*. 2019;20(1):158. doi:https://doi.org/10.3390/ijms20010158

20. Wang B, Han Y, Zhang Y, et al. Overcoming acquired resistance to cancer immune checkpoint therapy: potential strategies based on molecular mechanisms. *Cell & Bioscience*. 2023;13(1). doi:https://doi.org/10.1186/s13578-023-01073-9

21. Chae YK, Arya A, Iams W, et al. Current landscape and future of dual anti-CTLA4 and PD-1/PD-L1 blockade immunotherapy in cancer; lessons learned from clinical trials with melanoma and non-small cell lung cancer (NSCLC). *Journal for ImmunoTherapy of Cancer*. 2018;6(1). doi:https://doi.org/10.1186/s40425-018-0349-3

22. Rotte A. Combination of CTLA-4 and PD-1 blockers for treatment of cancer. *Journal of Experimental & Clinical Cancer Research*. 2019;38(1). doi:https://doi.org/10.1186/s13046-019-1259-z

23. Oxnard GR, Arcila ME, Chmielecki J, Ladanyi M, Miller VA, Pao W. New Strategies in Overcoming Acquired Resistance to Epidermal Growth Factor Receptor Tyrosine Kinase Inhibitors in Lung Cancer. *Clinical Cancer Research*. 2011;17(17):5530-5537. doi:https://doi.org/10.1158/1078-0432.ccr-10-2571

24. Zahavi DJ, Weiner LM. Targeting Multiple Receptors to Increase Checkpoint Blockade Efficacy. *International Journal of Molecular Sciences.* 2019;20(1):158. doi:https://doi.org/10.3390/ijms20010158

25. Mahesh Koirala, DiPaola M. Overcoming Cancer Resistance: Strategies and Modalities for Effective Treatment. *Biomedicines.* 2024;12(8):1801-1801. doi:https://doi.org/10.3390/biomedicines12081801

26. Bicak M, Cimen Bozkus C, Bhardwaj N. Checkpoint therapy in cancer treatment: progress, challenges, and future directions. *Journal of Clinical Investigation.* 2024;134(18). doi:https://doi.org/10.1172/jci184846

27. Bispecific Antibodies. Bccancer.bc.ca. Published 2019. Accessed November 21, 2024. http://www.bccancer.bc.ca/health-professionals/clinical-resources/chemotherapy-protocols/immunotherapy/bispecific-antibodies

28. Ordóñez-Reyes C, Garcia-Robledo JE, Chamorro DF, et al. Bispecific Antibodies in Cancer Immunotherapy: A Novel Response to an Old Question. *Pharmaceutics.* 2022;14(6):1243. doi:https://doi.org/10.3390/pharmaceutics14061243

29. Bmj.com. Published 2020. Accessed November 21, 2024. https://jitc.bmj.com/content/10/12/e005543

30. Li T, Wang X, Niu M, et al. Bispecific antibody targeting TGF-β and PD-L1 for synergistic cancer immunotherapy. *Frontiers in Immunology.* 2023;14. doi:https://doi.org/10.3389/fimmu.2023.1196970

31. Lakins MA, Koers A, Giambalvo R, et al. FS222, a CD137/PD-L1 Tetravalent Bispecific Antibody, Exhibits Low Toxicity and Antitumor Activity in Colorectal Cancer Models. *Clinical Cancer Research.* 2020;26(15):4154-4167. doi:https://doi.org/10.1158/1078-0432.ccr-19-2958

32. Lakins MA, Munoz-Olaya J, Veyssier C, et al. Abstract 1864: FS222, a tetravalent bispecific antibody targeting CD137 and PD-L1, is designed for optimal CD137 interactions resulting in potent T cell activation without toxicity. *Cancer Research.* 2021;81(13_Supplement):1864-1864. doi:https://doi.org/10.1158/1538-7445.am2021-1864

33. BiTE: The Future of Cancer Treatment through Clinical Trials - OHC. OHC - Oncology Hematology Care. Published May 30, 2023. https://ohcare.com/bite-clinical-trials/

34. Einsele H, Borghaei H, Orlowski RZ, et al. The BiTE (bispecific T-cell engager) platform: Development and future potential of a targeted immuno-oncology therapy across tumor types. *Cancer.* 2020;126(14):3192-3201. doi:https://doi.org/10.1002/cncr.32909

35. Hurwitz J, Haggstrom L, Lim E. Antibody–Drug Conjugates: Ushering in a New Era of Cancer Therapy. *Pharmaceutics.* 2023;15(8):2017-2017. doi:https://doi.org/10.3390/pharmaceutics15082017

36. Riccardi F, Michele Dal Bo, Paolo Macor, Toffoli G. A comprehensive overview on antibody-drug conjugates: from the conceptualization to cancer therapy. *Frontiers in*

Pharmacology. 2023;14. doi:https://doi.org/10.3389/fphar.2023.1274088

37. Zahavi DJ, Weiner LM. Targeting Multiple Receptors to Increase Checkpoint Blockade Efficacy. *International Journal of Molecular Sciences*. 2019;20(1):158. doi:https://doi.org/10.3390/ijms20010158

38. Han G, Chen G, Shen B, Li Y. Tim-3: An Activation Marker and Activation Limiter of Innate Immune Cells. *Frontiers in Immunology*. 2013;4. doi:https://doi.org/10.3389/fimmu.2013.00449

39. Tang W, Chen J, Ji T, Cong X. TIGIT, a novel immune checkpoint therapy for melanoma. *Cell Death & Disease*. 2023;14(7):1-9. doi:https://doi.org/10.1038/s41419-023-05961-3

40. Harjunpää H, Guillerey C. TIGIT as an emerging immune checkpoint. *Clinical & Experimental Immunology*. 2019;200(2). doi:https://doi.org/10.1111/cei.13407

41. Ge Z, Peppelenbosch MP, Sprengers D, Kwekkeboom J. TIGIT, the Next Step Towards Successful Combination Immune Checkpoint Therapy in Cancer. *Frontiers in Immunology*. 2021;12. doi:https://doi.org/10.3389/fimmu.2021.699895

42. Chu X, Tian W, Wang Z, Zhang J, Zhou R. Co-inhibition of TIGIT and PD-1/PD-L1 in Cancer Immunotherapy: Mechanisms and Clinical Trials. *Molecular Cancer*. 2023;22(1). doi:https://doi.org/10.1186/s12943-023-01800-3

43. Graydon CG, Mohideen S, Fowke KR. LAG3's Enigmatic Mechanism of Action. *Frontiers in Immunology*. 2021;11. doi:https://doi.org/10.3389/fimmu.2020.615317

44. Ruffo E, Wu RC, Bruno TC, Workman CJ, Vignali DAA. Lymphocyte-activation gene 3 (LAG3): The next immune checkpoint receptor. *Seminars in Immunology*. 2019;42:101305. doi:https://doi.org/10.1016/j.smim.2019.101305

45. Durham NM, Nirschl CJ, Jackson CM, et al. Lymphocyte Activation Gene 3 (LAG-3) Modulates the Ability of CD4 T-cells to Be Suppressed In Vivo. Kassiotis G, ed. *PLoS ONE*. 2014;9(11):e109080. doi:https://doi.org/10.1371/journal.pone.0109080

46. Luke JJ, Patel MR, Blumenschein GR, et al. The PD-1- and LAG-3-targeting bispecific molecule tebotelimab in solid tumors and hematologic cancers: a phase 1 trial. *Nature Medicine*. Published online October 19, 2023:1-11. doi:https://doi.org/10.1038/s41591-023-02593-0

47. Kreidieh FY, Tawbi HA. The introduction of LAG-3 checkpoint blockade in melanoma: immunotherapy landscape beyond PD-1 and CTLA-4 inhibition. *Therapeutic Advances in Medical Oncology*. 2023;15:17588359231186027. doi:https://doi.org/10.1177/17588359231186027

48. https://www.facebook.com/Drugscom. Opdualag (nivolumab and relatlimab-rmbw) FDA Approval History. Drugs.com. Published 2024. Accessed November 21, 2024. https://www.drugs.com/history/opdualag.html

49. Opdualag Approved to Treat Advanced Melanoma - National Cancer Institute. www.cancer.gov. Published April 6, 2022. https://www.cancer.gov/news-events/cancer-currents-blog/2022/fda-opdualag-melanoma-lag-3

50. Xu W, Dong J, Zheng Y, et al. Immune-Checkpoint Protein VISTA Regulates Antitumor Immunity by Controlling Myeloid Cell–Mediated Inflammation and Immunosuppression. 2019;7(9):1497-1510. doi:https://doi.org/10.1158/2326-6066.cir-18-0489

51. ElTanbouly MA, Croteau W, Noelle RJ, Lines JL. VISTA: A novel immunotherapy target for normalizing innate and adaptive immunity. *Seminars in Immunology*. 2019;42:101308. doi:https://doi.org/10.1016/j.smim.2019.101308

52. Noelle RJ, J. Louise Lines, Lewis LD, et al. Clinical and research updates on the VISTA immune checkpoint: immuno-oncology themes and highlights. *Frontiers in oncology*. 2023;13. doi:https://doi.org/10.3389/fonc.2023.1225081

53. Hashmi A. VISTA Emerges as a Promising Immunotherapy Target in Cancer. *wwwtargetedonccom*. 2022;11. https://www.targetedonc.com/view/vista-emerges-as-a-promising-immunotherapy-target-in-cancer

54. Zhang RJ, Kim TK. VISTA-mediated immune evasion in cancer. *Experimental & Molecular Medicine*. Published online November 1, 2024. doi:https://doi.org/10.1038/s12276-024-01336-6

55. Xu Y, Gao Z, Hu R, et al. PD-L2 glycosylation promotes immune evasion and predicts anti-EGFR efficacy. *Journal for immunotherapy of cancer.* 2021;9(10):e002699. doi:https://doi.org/10.1136/jitc-2021-002699

56. Arrieta O, Montes-Servín E, Hernandez-Martinez JM, et al. Expression of PD-1/PD-L1 and PD-L2 in peripheral T-cells from non-small cell lung cancer patients. *Oncotarget.* 2017;8(60). doi:https://doi.org/10.18632/oncotarget.22025

57. Wang B, Pei J, Xu S, Liu J, Yu J. Recent advances in mRNA cancer vaccines: meeting challenges and embracing opportunities. *Frontiers in Immunology.* 2023;14. doi:https://doi.org/10.3389/fimmu.2023.1246682

58. College R. An update on mRNA cancer vaccines. Rcpath.org. Published 2021. https://www.rcpath.org/resource-report/an-update-on-mrna-cancer-vaccines.html

59. Personalised mRNA vaccines: a revolutionary new approach in melanoma treatment. www.gavi.org. https://www.gavi.org/vaccineswork/personalised-mrna-vaccines-revolutionary-new-approach-melanoma-treatment

60. Winstead E. How mRNA Vaccines Might Help Treat Cancer. National Cancer Institute. Published January 20, 2022. https://www.cancer.gov/news-events/cancer-currents-blog/2022/mrna-vaccines-to-treat-cancer

61. Hellgren F, Rosdahl A, Cerveira RA, et al. Modulation of innate immune response to mRNA vaccination after SARS-CoV-2 infection or sequential vaccination in humans. *JCI*

Insight. 2024;9(9). doi:https://doi.org/10.1172/jci.insight.175401

62. Verbeke R, Hogan MJ, Loré K, Pardi N. Innate immune mechanisms of mRNA vaccines. *Immunity.* 2022;55(11):1993-2005. doi:https://doi.org/10.1016/j.immuni.2022.10.014
63. Wang B, Pei J, Xu S, Liu J, Yu J. Recent advances in mRNA cancer vaccines: meeting challenges and embracing opportunities. *Frontiers in Immunology.* 2023;14. doi:https://doi.org/10.3389/fimmu.2023.1246682
64. Yang R, Cui J. Advances and applications of RNA vaccines in tumor treatment. *Molecular Cancer.* 2024;23(1). doi:https://doi.org/10.1186/s12943-024-02141-5
65. Philpott J. mRNA Covid-19 vaccines may boost cancer immunotherapy effectiveness. Clinical Trials Arena. Published September 30, 2024. Accessed November 21, 2024. https://www.clinicaltrialsarena.com/news/mrna-covid-19-vaccines-may-boost-cancer-immunotherapy-effectiveness/
66. Perlmutter Cancer Center Clinical Trial Tests Personalized mRNA Vaccine for Treating Metastatic Melanoma. NYU Langone News. Published 2024. Accessed November 21, 2024. https://nyulangone.org/news/perlmutter-cancer-center-clinical-trial-tests-personalized-mrna-vaccine-treating-metastatic-melanoma
67. Personalised mRNA vaccines: a revolutionary new approach in melanoma treatment. www.gavi.org.

https://www.gavi.org/vaccineswork/personalised-mrna-vaccines-revolutionary-new-approach-melanoma-treatment

68. World S. Freeman Hospital first in the world to administer "anti-cancer injection" - Newcastle Hospitals NHS Foundation Trust. Newcastle Hospitals NHS Foundation Trust. Published March 21, 2024. Accessed November 21, 2024. https://www.newcastle-hospitals.nhs.uk/news/freeman-hospital-first-in-the-world-to-administer-anti-cancer-injection/
69. TIMESOFINDIA.COM. In a first, England to roll out seven-minute cancer treatment jab; know how it works. The Times of India. Published August 30, 2023. Accessed November 21, 2024. https://timesofindia.indiatimes.com/life-style/health-fitness/health-news/in-a-first-england-to-roll-out-seven-minute-cancer-treatment-jab-know-how-it-works/articleshow/103211725.cms
70. Sonika Nitin Nimje. England to be offer world-first seven-minute cancer treatment injection. @bsindia. Published August 31, 2023. https://www.business-standard.com/world-news/england-to-be-offer-world-first-seven-minute-cancer-treatment-injection-123083100553_1.html
71. FDA approves first subcutaneous anti-PD-L1 cancer immunotherapy. Healio.com. Published September 13, 2024. Accessed November 21, 2024. https://www.healio.com/news/hematology-oncology/20240913/fda-approves-first-subcutaneous-antipdl1-cancer-immunotherapy

72. National Cancer Institute. Atezolizumab - NCI. www.cancer.gov. Published May 20, 2016. https://www.cancer.gov/about-cancer/treatment/drugs/atezolizumab

73. NHS England to offer world-first seven-minute cancer treatment injection - PMLiVE. PMLiVE. Published August 30, 2023. Accessed November 21, 2024. https://pmlive.com/pharma_news/nhs_england_to_offer_world-first_seven-minute_cancer_treatment_injection_1496949/

74. Brooks N. The MHRA's International Recognition Procedure: new medicine approval in 2–4 months. Somerville Partners. Published November 17, 2023. https://somerville-partners.com/international-recognition-procedure-new-medicine-approval-in-2-4-months/

75. Nicolle L. NHS becomes first health system to roll out seven-minute anti-cancer injection. Pavilion Health Today - Supporting healthcare professionals to deliver the best patient care. Published August 30, 2023. Accessed November 21, 2024. https://pavilionhealthtoday.com/gm/nhs-becomes-first-health-system-to-roll-out-seven-minute-anti-cancer-injection/

76. Cunningham J, Drake K. Merck Announces Phase 3 Trial of Subcutaneous Pembrolizumab With Berahyaluronidase Alfa Met Primary Endpoints - Merck.com. Merck.com. Published November 22, 2024. https://www.merck.com/news/merck-announces-phase-3-

trial-of-subcutaneous-pembrolizumab-with-berahyaluronidase-alfa-met-primary-endpoints/

77. Inoue Y. Subcutaneous delivery of immune checkpoint inhibitors: new route replacing intravenous administration? *Translational Lung Cancer Research.* 2024;13(4):947-951. doi:https://doi.org/10.21037/tlcr-24-63

78. Scott R. Subcutaneous Pembrolizumab Plus Chemo Meets Pharmacokinetic End Points in NSCLC. OncLive. Published November 19, 2024. Accessed December 3, 2024. https://www.onclive.com/view/subcutaneous-pembrolizumab-plus-chemo-meets-pharmacokinetic-end-points-in-nsclc

Chapter 9

1. Chen Z, Shi T, Zhang L, et al. Mammalian drug efflux transporters of the ATP binding cassette (ABC) family in multidrug resistance: A review of the past decade. *Cancer Letters.* 2016;370(1):153-164. doi:https://doi.org/10.1016/j.canlet.2015.10.010

2. Kopcho N, Chang G, Komives EA. Dynamics of ABC Transporter P-glycoprotein in Three Conformational States. *Scientific Reports.* 2019;9(1):15092. doi:https://doi.org/10.1038/s41598-019-50578-2

3. Robey RW, Pluchino KM, Hall MD, Fojo AT, Bates SE, Gottesman MM. Revisiting the role of ABC transporters in multidrug-resistant cancer. *Nature Reviews Cancer.* 2018;18(7):452-464. doi:https://doi.org/10.1038/s41568-018-0005-8

4. Oup.com. Published 2024. Accessed November 21, 2024. https://academic.oup.com/jnci/article/107/9/djv222/901129?login=false#google_vignette

5. Bethune G, Bethune D, Ridgway N, Xu Z. Epidermal growth factor receptor (EGFR) in lung cancer: an overview and update. *Journal of Thoracic Disease.* 2010;2(1):48. https://pmc.ncbi.nlm.nih.gov/articles/PMC3256436/

6. Gao X, Zhang M, Tang Y, Liang X. Cancer cell dormancy: mechanisms and implications of cancer recurrence and metastasis. *OncoTargets and Therapy.* 2017;Volume 10:5219-5228. doi:https://doi.org/10.2147/ott.s140854

7. Freeborn J. Chemotherapy may sometimes reactivate dormant cancer cells. Medicalnewstoday.com. Published September 19, 2023. Accessed November 21, 2024. https://www.medicalnewstoday.com/articles/chemotherapy-may-sometimes-reactivate-dormant-cancer-cells

8. Wu P, Gao W, Su M, et al. Adaptive Mechanisms of Tumor Therapy Resistance Driven by Tumor Microenvironment. *Frontiers in Cell and Developmental Biology.* 2021;9. doi:https://doi.org/10.3389/fcell.2021.641469

9. Edwardson DW, Boudreau J, Mapletoft J, Lanner C, Kovala AT, Parissenti AM. Inflammatory cytokine production in tumor cells upon chemotherapy drug exposure or upon selection for drug resistance. Ahmad A, ed. *PLOS ONE.* 2017;12(9):e0183662. doi:https://doi.org/10.1371/journal.pone.0183662

10. Sun X, Yu Q. Intra-tumor heterogeneity of cancer cells and its implications for cancer treatment. *Acta Pharmacologica Sinica.* 2015;36(10):1219-1227. doi:https://doi.org/10.1038/aps.2015.92

11. Mokhtari RB, Homayouni TS, Baluch N, et al. Combination Therapy in Combating Cancer. *Oncotarget.* 2017;8(23). doi:https://doi.org/10.18632/oncotarget.16723

12. Palmer AC, Sorger PK. Combination Cancer Therapy Can Confer Benefit via Patient-to-Patient Variability without Drug Additivity or Synergy. *Cell.* 2017;171(7):1678-1691.e13. doi:https://doi.org/10.1016/j.cell.2017.11.009

13. Hu C, Mi W, Li F, et al. Optimizing drug combination and mechanism analysis based on risk pathway crosstalk in pan cancer. *Scientific Data.* 2024;11(1):74. doi:https://doi.org/10.1038/s41597-024-02915-y

14. Zhu L, Jiang M, Wang H, et al. A narrative review of tumor heterogeneity and challenges to tumor drug therapy. *Annals of Translational Medicine.* 2021;9(16):1351. doi:https://doi.org/10.21037/atm-21-1948

15. Mroz EA, Rocco JW. The challenges of tumor genetic diversity. *Cancer.* 2017;123(6):917-927. doi:https://doi.org/10.1002/cncr.30430

16. Shahid K, Khalife M, Dabney R, Phan AT. Immunotherapy and targeted therapy—the new roadmap in cancer treatment. *Annals of Translational Medicine.* 2019;7(20):595-595. doi:https://doi.org/10.21037/atm.2019.05.58

17. Ayoub NM. Editorial: Novel Combination Therapies for the Treatment of Solid Cancers. *Frontiers in Oncology*. 2021;11. doi:https://doi.org/10.3389/fonc.2021.708943

18. Bianchi G, Albanell J, Eiermann W, et al. Pilot Trial of Trastuzumab Starting with or after the Doxorubicin Component of a Doxorubicin plus Paclitaxel Regimen for Women with HER2-Positive Advanced Breast Cancer. *Clinical Cancer Research*. 2003;9(16):5944-5951. Accessed November 21, 2024. https://aacrjournals.org/clincancerres/article/9/16/5944/202175/Pilot-Trial-of-Trastuzumab-Starting-with-or-after

19. Espelin CW, Leonard SC, Geretti E, Wickham TJ, Hendriks BS. Dual HER2 Targeting with Trastuzumab and Liposomal-Encapsulated Doxorubicin (MM-302) Demonstrates Synergistic Antitumor Activity in Breast and Gastric Cancer. *Cancer Research*. 2016;76(6):1517-1527. doi:https://doi.org/10.1158/0008-5472.can-15-1518

20. Habib TN, Altonsy MO, Ghanem SA, Salama MS, Hosny MA. Optimizing combination therapy in prostate cancer: mechanistic insights into the synergistic effects of Paclitaxel and Sulforaphane-induced apoptosis. *BMC Molecular and Cell Biology*. 2024;25:5. doi:https://doi.org/10.1186/s12860-024-00501-z

21. Mason-Osann E, Pomeroy AE, Palmer AC, Mettetal JT. SYNERGISTIC DRUG COMBINATIONS PROMOTE THE DEVELOPMENT OF RESISTANCE IN ACUTE MYELOID LEUKEMIA. *Blood cancer discovery*.

Published online January 17, 2024. doi:https://doi.org/10.1158/2643-3230.bcd-23-0067

22. Hanna K, Mayden K. Chemotherapy treatment considerations in metastatic breast cancer. *Journal of the Advanced Practitioner in Oncology*. 2021;12(2). doi:https://doi.org/10.6004/jadpro.2021.12.2.11

23. Bischoff J, Ignatov A. The Role of Targeted Agents in the Treatment of Metastatic Breast Cancer. *Breast Care*. 2010;5(3):134-141. doi:https://doi.org/10.1159/000314996

24. Von Hoff DD, Ervin T, Arena FP, et al. Increased survival in pancreatic cancer with nab-paclitaxel plus gemcitabine. *The New England Journal of Medicine*. 2013;369(18):1691-1703. doi:https://doi.org/10.1056/NEJMoa1304369

25. Wu M, Huang X, Chen M, Zhang Y. Administration sequences in single-day chemotherapy regimens for breast cancer: a comprehensive review from a practical perspective. *Frontiers in Oncology*. 2024;14. doi:https://doi.org/10.3389/fonc.2024.1353067

26. Timing and Sequence Critical for Immunotherapy Combination. Cancer.gov. Published October 3, 2017. Accessed November 21, 2024. https://www.cancer.gov/news-events/cancer-currents-blog/2017/combining-checkpoint-inhibitors

27. Combination Cancer Therapy - Cancer. Merck Manuals Consumer Version. https://www.merckmanuals.com/home/cancer/prevention-and-treatment-of-cancer/combination-cancer-therapy

28. Abd El-Hafeez T, Shams MY, Elshaier YAMM, Farghaly HM, Hassanien AE. Harnessing machine learning to find synergistic combinations for FDA-approved cancer drugs. *Scientific Reports.* 2024;14(1):2428. doi:https://doi.org/10.1038/s41598-024-52814-w

29. Li R, Liu M, Yang Z, Li J, Gao Y, Tan R. Proteolysis-Targeting Chimeras (PROTACs) in Cancer Therapy: Present and Future. *Molecules.* 2022;27(24):8828. doi:https://doi.org/10.3390/molecules27248828

30. Burke MR, Smith AR, Zheng G. Overcoming Cancer Drug Resistance Utilizing PROTAC Technology. *Frontiers in Cell and Developmental Biology.* 2022;10. doi:https://doi.org/10.3389/fcell.2022.872729

31. PROTACtion against resistance of commonly used anti-cancer drug | Center for Cancer Research. Cancer.gov. Published 2023. Accessed November 21, 2024. https://ccr.cancer.gov/news/article/protaction-against-resistance-of-commonly-used-anti-cancer-drug

32. Yedla P, Babalghith AO, Andra VV, Syed R. PROTACs in the Management of Prostate Cancer. *Molecules.* 2023;28(9):3698. doi:https://doi.org/10.3390/molecules28093698

33. Petrylak D. Overcoming Hormone Resistance: ARV-766 in Advanced Prostate Cancer - Daniel Petrylak. UroToday. Published 2024. Accessed November 21, 2024. https://www.urotoday.com/video-lectures/crawford-s-corner-video-channel/video/4237-overcoming-hormone-resistance-arv-766-in-advanced-prostate-cancer-daniel-petrylak.html

34. Troup RI, Fallan C, Baud MGJ. Current strategies for the design of PROTAC linkers: a critical review. *Exploration of Targeted Anti-tumor Therapy.* 2020;1(5):273-312. doi:https://doi.org/10.37349/etat.2020.00018

35. Liu Z, Hu M, Yang Y, et al. An overview of PROTACs: a promising drug discovery paradigm. *Molecular Biomedicine.* 2022;3(1). doi:https://doi.org/10.1186/s43556-022-00112-0

36. Li X, Song Y. Proteolysis-targeting chimera (PROTAC) for targeted protein degradation and cancer therapy. *Journal of Hematology & Oncology.* 2020;13(1). doi:https://doi.org/10.1186/s13045-020-00885-3

37. Rutherford KA, McManus KJ. PROTACs: Current and Future Potential as a Precision Medicine Strategy to Combat Cancer. *Molecular cancer therapeutics.* 2024;23(4):454-463. doi:https://doi.org/10.1158/1535-7163.mct-23-0747

38. Arvinas unveils PROTAC structures. Chemical & Engineering News. https://cen.acs.org/pharmaceuticals/drug-discovery/Arvinas-unveils-PROTAC-structures/99/i14

39. Flanagan J, Qian Y, Gough S, et al. Abstract P5-04-18: ARV-471, an oral estrogen receptor PROTAC degrader for breast cancer. *Cancer Research.* 2019;79(4_Supplement):P5-0418. doi:https://doi.org/10.1158/1538-7445.SABCS18-P5-04-18

40. Vitamin D and Cancer Prevention. National Cancer Institute. Published 2017. https://www.cancer.gov/about-cancer/causes-prevention/risk/diet/vitamin-d-fact-sheet

41. The Power of Vitamin D: From Osteoporosis to Cancer - Medical Frontiers. NHK WORLD. Published 2024. Accessed November 21, 2024. https://www3.nhk.or.jp/nhkworld/en/shows/2050152/

42. Manson JE, Cook NR, Lee I-Min, et al. Vitamin D Supplements and Prevention of Cancer and Cardiovascular Disease. *New England Journal of Medicine.* 2019;380(1):33-44. doi:https://doi.org/10.1056/nejmoa1809944

43. Amirhossein Ghaseminejad-Raeini, Ghaderi A, Sharafi A, et al. Immunomodulatory actions of vitamin D in various immune-related disorders: a comprehensive review. *Frontiers in Immunology.* 2023;14. doi:https://doi.org/10.3389/fimmu.2023.950465

44. Sassi F, Tamone C, D'Amelio P. Vitamin D: Nutrient, Hormone, and Immunomodulator. *Nutrients.* 2018;10(11):1656. doi:https://doi.org/10.3390/nu10111656

45. Jeon SM, Shin EA. Exploring vitamin D metabolism and function in cancer. *Experimental & Molecular Medicine.* 2018;50(4). doi:https://doi.org/10.1038/s12276-018-0038-9

Chapter 10

1. Mullard A. PD1 agonist antibody passes first phase II trial for autoimmune disease. *Nature Reviews Drug Discovery.*

2023;22(7):526-526. doi:https://doi.org/10.1038/d41573-023-00087-9

2. Tuttle J, Drescher E, Jesus Abraham Simón-Campos, et al. A Phase 2 Trial of Peresolimab for Adults with Rheumatoid Arthritis. *The New England journal of medicine.* 2023;388(20):1853-1862. doi:https://doi.org/10.1056/nejmoa2209856

3. Gouda NA, Elkamhawy A, Cho J. Emerging Therapeutic Strategies for Parkinson's Disease and Future Prospects: A 2021 Update. *Biomedicines.* 2022;10(2):371. doi:https://doi.org/10.3390/biomedicines10020371

4. Adamu A, Li S, Gao F, Xue G. The role of neuroinflammation in neurodegenerative diseases: current understanding and future therapeutic targets. *Frontiers in aging neuroscience.* 2024;16(14). doi:https://doi.org/10.3389/fnagi.2024.1347987

5. Baruch K, Deczkowska A, Rosenzweig N, et al. PD-1 immune checkpoint blockade reduces pathology and improves memory in mouse models of Alzheimer's disease. *Nature Medicine.* 2016;22(2):135-137. doi:https://doi.org/10.1038/nm.4022

6. Curnock AP, Bossi G, Kumaran J, et al. Cell-targeted PD-1 agonists that mimic PD-L1 are potent T cell inhibitors. *JCI Insight.* 2021;6(20). doi:https://doi.org/10.1172/jci.insight.152468

7. Wykes MN, Lewin SR. Immune checkpoint blockade in infectious diseases. *Nature Reviews Immunology.* 2017;18(2):91-104. doi:https://doi.org/10.1038/nri.2017.112

8. Ferrando-Martinez S, Snell Bennett A, Lino E, et al. Functional Exhaustion of HBV-Specific CD8 T Cells Impedes PD-L1 Blockade Efficacy in Chronic HBV Infection. *Frontiers in Immunology*. 2021;12(12). doi:https://doi.org/10.3389/fimmu.2021.648420

9. Gambichler T, Reuther J, Scheel CH, Becker JC. On the use of immune checkpoint inhibitors in patients with viral infections including COVID-19. *Journal for ImmunoTherapy of Cancer*. 2020;8(2):e001145. doi:https://doi.org/10.1136/jitc-2020-001145

10. Colston E, Grasela D, Gardiner D, et al. An open-label, multiple ascending dose study of the anti-CTLA-4 antibody ipilimumab in viremic HIV patients. Landay A, ed. *PLOS ONE*. 2018;13(6):e0198158. doi:https://doi.org/10.1371/journal.pone.0198158

11. Gardiner D, Lalezari J, Lawitz E, et al. A Randomized, Double-Blind, Placebo-Controlled Assessment of BMS-936558, a Fully Human Monoclonal Antibody to Programmed Death-1 (PD-1), in Patients with Chronic Hepatitis C Virus Infection. Ahlenstiel G, ed. *PLoS ONE*. 2013;8(5):e63818. doi:https://doi.org/10.1371/journal.pone.0063818

12. Philips EA, Liu J, Audun Kvalvaag, et al. Transmembrane domain–driven PD-1 dimers mediate T cell inhibition. *Science Immunology*. 2024;9(93). doi:https://doi.org/10.1126/sciimmunol.ade6256

www.ingramcontent.com/pod-product-compliance
Lightning Source LLC
Chambersburg PA
CBHW070804280326
41934CB00012B/3056

* 9 7 9 8 9 9 2 1 5 8 3 0 4 *